The Johns Hopkins Hospital
2002 Guide to
MEDICAL CARE
of
PATIENTS WITH
HIV INFECTION

Tenth Edition

The Johns Hopkins Hospital 2002 Guide to
MEDICAL CARE
of
PATIENTS WITH HIV INFECTION
Tenth Edition

John G. Bartlett, M.D.

Professor of Medicine
Chief, Division of Infectious Diseases
Director, AIDS Service
Johns Hopkins University School of Medicine
Baltimore, Maryland

 LIPPINCOTT WILLIAMS & WILKINS

A **Wolters Kluwer** Company

Philadelphia · Baltimore · New York · London
Buenos Aires · Hong Kong · Sydney · Tokyo

Editor: Jonathan Pine
Managing Editor: Jennifer Kullgren
Developmental Editor: Raymond E. Reter
Marketing Manager: Julie Sikora
Purchasing Manager, Clinical and Healthcare: Jennifer Jett
Compositor: Maryland Composition
Printer: Vicks Lithograph & Printing

© 2001 by LIPPINCOTT WILLIAMS & WILKINS
530 Walnut Street
Philadelphia, PA 19106 USA
LWW.com

Printed in the USA

ISBN 0-7817-3427-4

First Edition, 1991
Second Edition, 1992
Third Edition, 1993
Fourth Edition, 1994

Fifth Edition, 1995
Sixth Edition, 1996
Seventh Edition, 1997
Eighth Edition, 1998

Ninth Edition, 2000
Tenth Edition, 2001

Care has been taken to confirm the accuracy of the information presented and to describe generally accepted practices. However, the authors, editors, and publisher are not responsible for errors or omissions or for any consequences from application of the information in this book and make no warranty, expressed or implied, with respect to the currency, completeness, or accuracy of the contents of the publication. Application of this information in a particular situation remains the professional responsibility of the practitioner.

The authors, editors, and publisher have exerted every effort to ensure that drug selection and dosage set forth in this text are in accordance with current recommendations and practice at the time of publication. However, in view of ongoing research, changes in government regulations, and the constant flow of information relating to drug therapy and drug reactions, the reader is urged to check the package insert for each drug for any change in indications and dosage and for added warnings and precautions. This is particularly important when the recommended agent is a new or infrequently employed drug.

Some drugs and medical devices presented in this publication have Food and Drug Administration (FDA) clearance for limited use in restricted research settings. It is the responsibility of the health care provider to ascertain the FDA status of each drug or device planned for use in their clinical practice.

01 02
1 2 3 4 5 6 7 8 9 10

PREFACE

The purpose of this publication is to provide guidelines for the care of patients with HIV infection. These recommendations reflect the policies of the AIDS Care Program at Johns Hopkins Hospital, where approximately 3000 patients with this infection are being followed. Recommendations for HIV care change frequently, so the care provider is cautioned that this guideline is dated August 2001. The tenth edition has been augmented by additional tables and extensive revision of the text reflecting dramatic changes in the prognosis of HIV owing to advances in the field and the incredible complexity of care that accompanies these advances. This edition includes guidelines for management of HIV/AIDS from the Department of Health and Human Services for 2001.

For updated information visit our website: www.hopkins-aids.edu

LIST OF TABLES AND FIGURES

FIGURES

CONTENTS

1—HIV Serology

Indications

Rapidly evolving improvements in medical care provide the incentive for increased serologic testing. The CDC suggests that hospitals in which seroprevalence rates exceed 1% or in which the case rate of AIDS exceeds 1/1000 discharges should offer serology as a routine admission laboratory test to persons aged 15–54 yr (NEJM 1992;327:445; MMWR 1993;42[RR-2]; Lancet 1996;348:176). Persons in high-risk categories are an obvious priority.

Informed Consent

Testing should be voluntary with appropriate counseling. Informed consent is required by law in 41 states, and some laboratories have policies that require the signature of the patient or the legal representative as a contingency for processing. An exception is that many states permit testing of the source with exposures to health care workers. Some areas offer anonymous testing in which all patient identifiers are removed. The usual charge for the test is $30–60; most state and local health departments offer HIV serology at no charge. There are 31 states that have required reporting of all persons with positive HIV serology. All states have mandatory reporting of AIDS cases.

Accuracy

Test results are reported as positive, negative, or indeterminate. The standard serologic test requires a positive enzyme-linked immunoabsorbent assay (ELISA) as a screening test and a positive Western blot for confirmation. The usual criteria by Western blot are plus gp 120/160 or gp 41 plus gp 120/160. Variations in diagnostic criteria and weak bands sometimes cause inconsistencies in reports, but this is unusual. CDC testing of 1400 clinical labs in 1990 showed sensitivity of 99.3% and specificity of 99.7% (MMWR 1990;39:380). The rate of <u>false-positive tests</u> in a low-prevalence population with both ELISA and

Western blot is about 1/135,000 or 0.0007% (NEJM 1988;319: 961; N Engl J Med 1993;328:1281).

The frequency of <u>false-negative results</u> in a high-prevalence population (IV drug users with a seroprevalence rate of 30%) is about 0.3% (JID 1993;168:327), and in a low-prevalence population (blood donors) it is about 0.001% (NEJM 1991;325:1, 593). The usual cause of false-negative tests is testing during the time between transmission and seroconversion, a period that usually averages 10–12 days (CID 1997;25:101; Am J Med 2000;160: 3286). Other causes of false-negative results are agammaglobulinemia or infection with strains that are antigenically distinctive (Lancet 1996;348:176) such as HIV-2 (JAMA 1992;267:2775; Ann Intern Med 1993;118:211) or the subtype O of HIV-1 (Lancet 1993;343:1393; MMWR 1996;45:561; Lancet 1994;344:1333). HIV-2 has been reported in 78 patients in the U.S. from 1987 through January 1998, most of whom immigrated from or acquired the disease in West Africa (MMWR 1995;44:603). Standard EIA screening assays used in the U.S. may include antigens to both HIV-1 and HIV-2; screening EIA tests for HIV-1 are positive in 70–80% of patients with HIV-2 infection, although Western blots are often indeterminant or negative (JAMA 1992;267:2775; Ann Intern Med 1993;118:211). Testing for HIV-2 is recommended for patients from countries where HIV-2 is prevalent and those who are needle-sharing or sexual partners of such patients, persons who received transfusions in the endemic area, or children born of infected women. These countries include Benin, Burkina Faso, Ghana, Guinea, Nigeria, Liberia, Sao Tome, Senegal, Togo, Cape Verde, Ivory Coast, Gambia, Guinea-Bissau, Mali, Mauritania, and Sierra Leone. Only one case of HIV infection involving subtype O has occurred in the U.S. through July 1996 (MMWR 1996;45:561). Type IV strains could also cause false-negative results, but there have been no cases of cases of this infection in the U.S. (JID 2000;181: 470). There are rare patients with persistently false-negative serologic tests (AIDS 1995;9:95; MMWR 1996;45:181; CID 1997; 25:98; CID 1997;25:101).

The most common cause of <u>indeterminate results</u> is a positive ELISA and a single band on a Western blot. This may reflect seroconversion in process, so the test should be repeated in 3–4 mo. Persons in low-risk categories with indeterminate test results are virtually never infected with either HIV-1 or HIV-2; repeat testing is likely to show persistence of indeterminant results, and the cause of this pattern is usually unknown (NEJM 1990;322:217). In view of the unnecessary anxiety evoked by knowledge of possible HIV infection, low-risk patients with indeterminate tests should be reassured that HIV infection is very unlikely, but the follow-up test is necessary to provide 100% assurance. When a non–antibody-dependent assay is necessary to confirm or clarify serologic assays, the preferred test is qualitative plasma HIV DNA PCR; this shows sensitivity of 97–98% and specificity of 98% (Ann Intern Med 1996;124:803).

Alternative Diagnostic Methods to Detect HIV

Alternative tests have been developed to increase access to testing (home test), to improve acceptability of testing (urine or salivary assays), and to reduce the time delay in availability of results.

Home Tests. The only FDA-approved home test is the Home Access Express Test (Home Access Health Corporation, Hoffman Estates, IL; 800-HIV-TEST). The Home Access Test is available in pharmacies at $35–50/test. Blood is obtained by lancet; one drop is placed on a filter strip, and this is mailed using an anonymous code for patient identity. Testing consists of a double EIA screening test and a confirming IFA test. Consumer telephones are for counseling, and results are available in ≥1 wk. Initial studies comparing home tests with standard serology show 100% sensitivity and 100% specificity (Arch Intern Med 1997;157:309). The advantage of this method is access to testing by some persons who are reluctant to use standard health care facilities. The main disadvantages are expense and concern for psychological reactions to results in a non-medical care environment.

Salivary test. OraSure (Epitope Co., Beaverton, OR; 888-ORA-SURE). A cotton pad is used to obtain saliva, which is placed in a vial and submitted to a lab for EIA and Western blot. A study of 3570 persons showed correct results compared with standard serology in 672 of 673 (99.9%) seropositives and 2893 of 2897 (99%) seronegatives (JAMA 1997;277:254). Results are available in 3 days by phone or fax. The cost is $99/three test kits.

Urine test. Calypte HIV-1 Urine EIA (Calypte Inc., 510-749-5153). This test uses urine for EIA screening or dot blot assay (Genie HIV-1/HIV-2, Genetic Systems) (Eur J Clin Microbiol Infect Dis 1996;15:810). Positive results require confirmation by standard serology. The test is supplied as a 192-test kit for $816 or a 480-test kit for $1920; this translates to $4/test.

Rapid Tests.   SUDS (Murex, Norcross, GA) is the only available FDA-approved rapid HIV serologic test. The test uses an EIA format and requires interpretation by a laboratory technician. The experience with the SUDS test in 6200 patients showed a sensitivity of 99.9–100% and specificity of 99.6% (J AIDS 1993;6:115; Am J Emerg Med 1991;9:416; Ann Intern Med 1996; 125:471). The cost for SUDS is $283 for 30 assays or $9/test. A single test requires two controls, so the total cost is $27 for one test and $36 for two tests. The advantage is that results are available in 10 min. Settings in which rapid screening results are highly desired are for 1) occupational exposures of healthcare workers and 2) clinical settings where immediate results are desired for patient counseling, especially when reliable follow-up is unlikely; examples are emergency rooms and STD clinics (Ann Intern Med 1996;125:471). Prior studies show that in many settings up to 40% of patients who receive routine serologic tests never return for results (Ann Intern Med 1996;125:471). The test is considered definitive if it is negative; patients with positive tests should have confirmation using standard serology. SUDS has two problems: 1) "Manufacturing problems" were announced October 17, 2000, and the time of availability is unknown. 2) The test must be performed by a lab technician. New tests are expected in 2001 that will accurately detect HIV using blood or saliva, and they are read by the provider, with results within 10–15 min (Ann Intern Med 1999;131:4810). These tests should remarkably improve HIV detection.

2—Epidemiology (Table 1)

Current estimates are that the seroprevalence of HIV in the U.S. is 0.3%, and 650,000–900,000 persons are living with HIV infection (JAMA 1996;276:126); about 335,000 are receiving HIV care. The total reported with AIDS (1993 definition) for 1981 through June 2001 was 774,467. Risk categories for 43,517 newly reported AIDS cases for FY 2000 follow: Gay men—33%, injection drug users—22%, both of these risks—4%, heterosexual contact—16%, perinatal transmission—0.5%, transfusion—0.6%, unknown/unspecified—25%.

Table 1. Seroprevalence of HIV in the United States

Category	Reference	Rate	Comment
Gay men	Am J Epidemiol 1987;126:568 J AIDS 1989;2:77 Science 1991;253:37 JAMA 1994;272:149 J AIDS 1995;9:514	14–50%	• Average in Multicenter AIDS Cohort Study (5000 participants) was 36% at entry with 0.5–1.0% annual seroconversion rate; higher seroconversion rates are reported in young gay men • Gay men accounted for 14,393 (33%) of newly reported cases of AIDS reported in adults and adolescents in FY 2000 and 348,657 of 745,103 (47%) of cumulative cases reported through June 2000
IV drug users	JAMA 1989;261:2677 J AIDS 1993;6:1049 AIDS 1994;8:263 Arch Intern Med 1995;155:1305	1–60%	• Review of 92 studies showed great variation by location: New York City 34–61%; New Jersey 17–29%; Boston 28%; Puerto Rico 45–59%; Detroit 8–12%; San Francisco 5–16%; Miami 5%; New Orleans 1%; Atlanta 10%; Denver 1–5%; Los Angeles 2–5%; Minnesota 1%. Annual seroconversion rate: Baltimore 4%; LA nil; Philadelphia 2.5% in clients of methadone clinics and 14% in active users not in treatment • IDU accounted for 9390 of 43,293 (22%) of newly reported cases of AIDS in adults and adolescents in FY 2000
Methadone clinic clients	N Engl J Med 1992;326:375	1–30%	• Eight city surveys with rates ranging from 0.7% (Seattle) to 28.6% (Newark); average is 9%
Hemophilia	JAMA 1985;253:3409 J AIDS 1994;7:279	Type A 70% Type B 35%	• Applies to hemophiliacs who received clotting factors before 1985. Hemophilia and 111 of 43,293 (0.2%) of newly reported AIDS cases in FY 2000 and a cumulative total of 5121 (1%) of 745,103 cases reported through June 2000

Group	Reference	Rate	Notes
Regular sex partners of HIV-infected persons	Arch Intern Med 1989;149:645 Am J Med 1988;85:472 JAMA 1991;266:1664 J AIDS 1993;6:497 Science 1995;270:1374 Am J Epidemiol 1997;146:350	0–58%	• Average is 20–25% for wives of hemophiliac men with HIV infection • Discordant couple study in the U.S. showed efficiency of transmission 8:1 greater for male → female, but this was not seen in the discordant couple study in Africa where the ratio was 1:1. Rate of transmission is highly dependent on viral load • Heterosexual transmission accounted for 6773 of 43,293 (16%) of newly reported adult cases in FY 2000
Women (age 18–59 yr)	Science 1995;270:1374 JAMA 1997;278:911	0.15%	• Women accounted for 10,469 of 43,293 (23%) newly reported AIDS cases in FY 2000. This compares with 534 of 8153 (7%) in 1985. Risk factors in reporting: IDU 2,795 (27%), heterosexual contact 4,114 (39%), no identified risk 3,420 (33%) • Great variation by location and confounding variable of IDU: Newark 57%; Washington DC 50%; Miami 19%; San Francisco 6%; Los Angeles 4%; Atlanta 1%; Las Vegas 0
Prostitutes	MMWR 1987;36:157 JAMA 1990;263:60	0–57%	
College students Childbearing women and perinatal transmission	N Engl J Med 1990;323:1538 JAMA 1991;265:1704 JAMA 1995;274:952	0.2% 0.15%	• Highest rates of HIV in pregnant woman were NYC 0.58%; Washington DC 0.55%; New Jersey 0.49%; Florida 0.45%
Pediatrics	MMWR 1996;45:1005	0.02%	• Perinatal transmission accounted for 224 of 43,517 (0.5%) newly reported AIDS cases in FY 2000 and a cumulative total of 8,804 of 753,907 (1%) of all AIDS cases reported through June 2000 • The number of perinatally acquired AIDS cases peaked in 1992 (905 cases) and decreased 75% in 2000

Table 1. (continued)

Category	Reference	Rate	Comment
STD clinic clients	STD 1992;19:235 J AIDS 1995;9:514 N Engl J Med 1992;326:375	0.5–11%	• Summary of 552,665 serologic tests in 80 STD clinics from 1988–92 showed HIV seroprevalence was 33% in gay men, 3% in heterosexual men, 2% in heterosexual women, and 10% in heterosexual injection drug users
Applicants to military	MMWR 1988;37:67 J AIDS 1990;3:1168 J AIDS 1995;10:177 JAMA 1991;265:1709	0.13%	• Annual seroconversion rate is 0.02–0.03%/yr
Transfusion recipients	N Engl J Med 1995;333:1721 N Engl J Med 1996;334:1685	0.02%	• Estimated 18–27 HIV transmissions/yr with blood transfusions in the U.S. • Transfusions accounted for 270 of newly reported AIDS cases in FY 2000 and hemophilia accounted for 111 newly reported AIDS cases in FY 2000 for an aggregate total of 0.9% • Risk is 1 per 450,000–660,000 units of screened blood
General population	Science 1991;253:37 MMWR 1990;30(RR-16) Science 1995;270:1374	0.4%	• Annual seroconversion rate in the U.S. based on assumption of 40,000 new infections/year is 0.016% • Annual seroconversion rate in young adult men is estimated at about 0.05%; new data in 2001 show annual seroconversion rates in gay men in some cities as high as 4.3%

3—Classification and Natural History

Classification

The current CDC classification system (Table 2) uses three ranges of CD4 cell counts (>500, $200-499$, and $<200/mm^3$) and a matrix of nine mutually exclusive categories. Category B includes most conditions previously classified as AIDS-related complex.

Natural History

Virologic Events and Immune Defense.
HIV infection involves the complex interplay of viral replication and immune defenses. Clinical expression in early-stage disease (acute retroviral syndrome) is similar to other acute viral infections; characteristic features in late-stage disease reflect immune destruction, largely because of loss of CD4 cells, which are critical factors for modulating host defenses.

The sequence of events is the following: HIV is transmitted across the mucocutaneous barrier with extension to regional lymph tissue (days) $\rightarrow$ massive viremia with maximum plasma HIV RNA levels 2–4 wk after transmission expressed as the acute HIV syndrome; this is accompanied by a high risk of HIV transmission to others, with sex or needle sharing exposure, widespread dissemination, and extensive involvement of lymph tissue (weeks) $\rightarrow$ immune response with partial control ascribed to cytotoxic T-cell response (primarily CD8 cells) that is regulated by HIV-specific CD4 cytokine response and then with seroconversion (weeks-months) $\rightarrow$ persistent HIV replication with relatively constant levels of HIV RNA viremia after the "set point" is established about 4 mo after HIV transmission. Once the set point is reached the CD4 cell count gradually decreases, and viral load only slightly increases (JID 1999;180:1018). The CD4 decline that averages $50/mm^3/yr$ over a mean of 8–10 yr $\rightarrow$ massive destruction of immune system with susceptibility to opportunistic pathogens and opportunistic tumors when the CD4 cell count reaches $<200/mm^3$ (N Engl J Med 1993;328:329) (Fig. 1).

The replication rate in chronically infected patients ranges from 18 to $460/mm^3$ and averages 10^{10} virions/day. The major

Table 2. AIDS Surveillance Case Definition for Adolescents and Adults: 1993 (MMWR 1992;41:1–9)

CD4 Cell Categories	Clinical Categories		
	A Asymptomatic, PGL, or Acute HIV Infection	B Symptomatic (Not A or C)[b]	C[a] AIDS Indicator Condition (1987)
1. >500/mm^3 (≥29%)	A1	B1	C1
2. 200–499/mm^3 (14–28%)	A2	B2	C2
3. <200/mm^3 (<14%)	A3	B3	C3

[a] All patients in categories A3, B3, C1–C3 are reported as AIDS based on prior AIDS indicator conditions (see below) and/or a CD4 cell count of <200/mm^3. AIDS indicator conditions include three new entries added to the 1987 case definition (MMWR 1987;36:15): Recurrent bacterial pneumonia, invasive cervical cancer, and pulmonary tuberculosis.

[b] Symptomatic conditions not included in category C that 1) are attributed to HIV infection or indicate a defect in cell-mediated immunity or 2) are conditions considered to have a clinical course or to require management that is complicated by HIV infection. Examples of B conditions include but are not limited to bacillary angiomatosis; thrush; vulvovaginal candidiasis that is persistent, frequent, or poorly responsive to therapy; cervical dysplasia (moderate or severe); cervical carcinoma in situ; constitutional symptoms such as fever (38.5° C) or diarrhea for >1 mo; oral hairy leukoplakia; herpes zoster involving two episodes of >1 dermatome; ITP; listeriosis; PID (especially if complicated by a tubo-ovarian abscess); peripheral neuropathy.

Indicator Conditions in Case Definition of AIDS

Candidiasis of esophagus, trachea, bronchi, or lungs
Cervical cancer, invasive[c,d]
Coccidioidomycosis, extrapulmonary[c]
Cryptococcosis, extrapulmonary
Cryptosporidiosis with diarrhea for >1 mo
Cytomegalovirus of any organ other than liver, spleen, or lymph nodes
Herpes simplex with mucocutaneous ulcer for >1 mo or bronchitis, pneumonitis, esophagitis
Histoplasmosis, extrapulmonary[c]
HIV-associated dementia[a]: disabling cognitive and/or motor dysfunction interfering with occupation or activities of daily living
HIV-associated wasting[c]: involuntary weight loss of >10% of baseline plus chronic diarrhea (≥2 loose stools/day for ≥30 days) or chronic weakness and documented enigmatic fever for ≥30 days
Isosporosis with diarrhea for >1 mo[c]
Kaposi's sarcoma in patient younger than 60 (or older than 60[c])
Lymphoma of brain in patient younger than 60 (or older than 60[c])
Lymphoma, non-Hodgkin's of B cell or unknown immunologic phenotype and histology showing small, noncleaved lymphoma or immunoblastic sarcoma
Mycobacterium avium or *M. kansasii*, disseminated[c]
Mycobacterium tuberculosis, disseminated[c]
Mycobacterium tuberculosis, pulmonary[c,d]
Pneumocystis carinii pneumonia
Pneumonia, recurrent-bacterial[c,d]
Progressive multifocal leukoencephalopathy
Salmonella septicemia (nontyphoid), recurrent[c]
Toxoplasmosis of internal organ

[c] Requires positive HIV serology.
[d] Added in the revised case definition 1993.

target of HIV is CD4 cells, and cell destruction represents the effect of viral clearance by cytotoxic T lymphocytes (CTL) or "killer cells" (Nature 1993;366:22). Current estimates are that the average healthy adult harbors 10^{12} CD4 cells; approximately 10–25% of the CD4 population is infected early during HIV infection, and HIV infection results in destruction of about 10^9 CD4 cells/day. These data indicate that 30% of the total body HIV burden turns over daily, and 6–7% of the CD4 cells turn over daily. These data are averages; kinetics of HIV and CD4 cells in individual patients are highly variable.

The course of the infection without therapy averages about 10 yr from the time of initial infection to an AIDS-defining diagnosis. In some patients, the rate of CD4 cell loss is rampant with counts of $<200/mm^3$ within 2 yr; at the other extreme are "chronic nonprogressors"—defined as patients with HIV infection for >8 yr and CD4 counts of $>500/mm^3$, with no antiviral treatment (Lancet 1993;340:863). Sequential analysis of two cohorts followed from the time of seroconversion show a mean duration to CD4 counts of $<500/mm^3$ of 48 mo (Ann Intern Med 1996;125:257). Some patients have an AIDS-defining diagnosis within 18 mo after seroconversion. In the MACS cohort, 20 of 1800 (0.9%) had no significant decline in CD4 counts despite HIV infection for 14 yr with no antiretroviral therapy. These variations in course are largely dependent on the cytotoxic T cell (CD8 cell) response, which is ultimately dependent on competency of CD4 cells that regulate CD8 cells with HIV-specific CD4 cell responses and cytokines (Science 1997;278:1447). The problem is the rapid consumption of CD4 cells by rapidly replicating HIV. The implication of these observations is that control of HIV replication in early stage disease (acute HIV syndrome) by natural defenses or HAART may lead to "long term nonprogression." Other factors that may influence the rate of progression follow:

- Defective virus (Lancet 1992;340:863): Rare
- Genetic susceptibility of receptor sites (Nature Med 1996; 2:966)
- Age: Duration of survival is inversely correlated with age (Lancet 1996;347:1573; Lancet 2000;355:1131). Note that

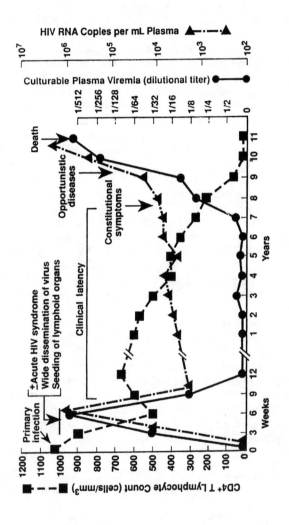

Figure 1. Typical course of HIV infection without therapy. The initial event is the acute retroviral syndrome accompanied by a decline in CD4 cell count (*squares*), high-level cultivable HIV plasma viremia (*circles*), and high plasma concentrations of HIV RNA (*triangles*) that reach zenith levels of 2–40 million copies/mL (JID 1999;180:1018). Clinical symptoms usually resolve spontaneously in 1–3 wk; this recovery is accompanied by a rapid decline in plasma viremia, reflecting CTL response (Science 1996;272:505; Science 1997;278:1447). The CD4 cell count may return toward baseline, although some studies show no rebound (Ann Intern Med 1996;125:257) and then show a linear decline that averages 50/mm^3/yr. The subsequent course generally shows a prolonged period of clinical latency that is accompanied by high rates of HIV replication with an average of approximately 10^{10} new virions/day. Plasma concentrations of HIV RNA predict the course (about 10^3/mL for slow progressors and $>10^5$/mL for rapid progressors) (Ann Intern Med 1997;126:946). The CD4 cell count decline (CD4 slope) is often accelerated during late-stage disease as indicated by the ''inflection point'' of the CD4 slope, and this is accompanied by increased levels of HIV RNA. A CD4 cell count of 200/mm^3 is generally regarded as the threshold at which patients become vulnerable to opportunistic infections. The median time to an AIDS-defining complication after reaching 200/mm^3 is 18–24 mo; the median survival after a CD4 count of 200/mm^3 is 3.1 yr; and the median survival after an AIDS-defining complication is 1.3 yr. (This is without antiretroviral therapy.) With no therapy directed against HIV and no PCP prophylaxis, the average time from viral transmission to an AIDS-defining diagnosis is about 10 yr. Data provided for the CD4 cell decline are averages based on natural history studies in the Multicenter AIDS Cohort Study (MACS) (JID 1993;168:149; J AIDS 1995;8:66). There is substantial individual variation; some patients have a rapid decline in CD4 cell counts after acute retroviral syndrome, and 5–15% are considered chronic nonprogressors with CD4 cell counts exceeding 500/mm^3 for more than 8 yr (J AIDS 1995;8:496). Given comparable care, there is no significant difference in rates of progression based on sex, race, or risk category. Variations in rates of progression in untreated adults correlate primarily with host defense, especially CTL response that is regulated by the HIV-specific CD4 cell response (Science 1996;271:324; PNAS 1997;94:254; Science 1997;278:1447). (Figure 1 is reproduced with permission from Ann Intern Med 1996;124:654; JID 1999;180:1018.)

other demographic characteristics (gender, race, risk, etc) do not seem to influence rates of progression
• Major histocompatibility genes (Nature Med 1996;4:405; Hosp Pract 1998;33:53)
• Plasma level of HIV RNA after the set point is established (Science 1996;272:1167; Ann Intern Med 1997;126:946)
• CTL response appears to be the cortical determinant of viral load set point and rate of progression (Science 1997;278: 1447)

Medical interventions that are associated with a significant increase in survival:

1. Antiretroviral therapy (NEJM 1998;338:853; Lancet 1998; 252:1725)
2. *P. carinii* prophylaxis (JAMA 1988;259:118)
3. *M. avium* prophylaxis (N Engl J Med 1996;335:384)
4. Care by a physician with HIV experience (NEJM 1996;334: 701)

Viral transmission. The efficiency of HIV transmission with discordant couples without antiviral therapy or condoms is estimated to be about 0.2% (Lancet 357:1149, 2001). This estimate is based on a longitudinal survey of discordant couples in Uganda; the actual frequency of transmission was 1/558 acts of sexual intercourse. The risk with a needlestick injury from an HIV-infected source is about 0.3% or about 1/300 (Ann Intern Med 1990;113:740). The rate for perinatal transmission is about 23% with vaginal delivery (NEJM 1996;335:1621). All of these rates are highly correlated with the viral load in the source (NEJM 1999;341:394; Lancet 2001;357:1149; AIDS 2001;15:621; JID 2001;183:206).

Acute HIV infection. This illness generally occurs 1–3 wk after an exposure such as a needle-stick injury in a health care worker or sexual exposure (Ann Intern Med 1996;125:257; Ann Intern Med 1993;118:913; JID 1994;168:1490). The time to seroconversion after viral transmission has been reported as long as 10 mo in a health care worker with occupationally acquired

Table 3. Acute HIV Infection

Symptomatic disease: 50–89%
Frequency of correct diagnosis with medical consultation: 25%
Incubation period (HIV exposure to onset of symptoms): 2–6 wk
Symptoms and signs

Fever	96%	Diarrhea	32%
Adenopathy	74%	Nausea or vomiting	27%
Pharyngitis	70%	Hepatosplenomegaly	14%
Rash[a]	70%	Thrush	12%
Myalgias	54%	Neurologic symptoms[b]	12%
Headache	32%		

Duration of symptoms (mean): 1–3 wk
Laboratory tests: Plasma viremia with high titer (peak of 2–40 million copies/
    mL). HIV-1 serologic test negative or indeterminant

Adapted from JID 1993;168:1490; Ann Intern Med 1996;125:257; CID 1998;26:323; JID 1997;
176:112.
[a] Erythematous maculopapular rash involving the face, trunk, and extremities ± soles
and palms. There may be mucocutaneous ulcerations involving the mouth, esophagus,
or genitals.
[b] Includes aseptic meningitis, meningoencephalitis, peripheral neuropathy, facial
palsey. Guillain-Barré syndrome, brachial neuritis, cognitive impairment, or psychosis.

HIV (NEJM 1998;339:33). The frequency with which this syndrome is clinically expressed in patients who have sequential blood samplings documenting seroconversion is 80–90% (CID 1998;26:323 JID 1997;176:112; BMJ 1989;299:154). Clinical features (Table 3) are those of an infectious mononucleosis-like illness with fever, adenopathy, hepatosplenomegaly, sore throat, myalgias, morbilliform rash, mucocutaneous ulceration, diarrhea, and leukopenia with atypical lymphocytes (Ann Intern Med 1993;118:913; JID 1994;168:1490; Ann Intern Med 1996; 125:257; CID 1998; 26:323). Some patients have neurologic symptoms such as aseptic meningitis, Guillain-Barré syndrome, or acute psychosis. The five most common clinical features in the Seattle study were fever (mean 38.9° C), sore throat, fatigue, malaise, and weight loss (average 5 kg); 17% were hospitalized and 24% had signs of aseptic meningitis (Ann Intern Med 1996; 125:257). The febrile illness is self-limited, usually lasting 1–3 wk. Laboratory studies may show leukopenia and increased transaminase levels. Serologic tests for HIV are negative. The diagnosis is best established by p24 antigen (which is 100% specific and 80% sensitive) or viral load (which is 100% sensitive and 90% specific) (Ann Intern Med 2001;134:25). The usual test in primary HIV is plasma HIV RNA. There are false-positives with this assay but only at low titer; the usual titer expected is >50,000 copies/mL. This is an important issue because aggressive treatment of primary HIV infection may be the optimal time to influence the disease course (JID 2001;183:1466). Nevertheless, these patients have replication competent HIV in latently infected CD4 cells, suggesting that several years of treatment may be necessary even in this group that represents the most favorable prognosis based on early therapy (Science 1997; 278:291).

Seroconversion.   Seroconversion generally takes place 3–5 wk after transmission (JAMA 1998;280:1080; Am J Med 2000; 109:568). The CTL response precedes humoral response and is accompanied by a sharp reduction in plasma concentrations of HIV RNA copies (PNAS 1997;94:254) and resolution of symptoms of acute HIV infection.

Establishment of HIV RNA plasma level set point.   Plasma levels of HIV RNA are established at a set point that is relatively stable over several years characterized as "chronic asymptomatic HIV infection." During this time there is a gradual increase in mean HIV RNA levels averaging about 7%/yr (Ann Intern Med 1998;128:613) with occassional blips reflecting antigenic stimuli (intercurrent illness or immunizations) (Ann Intern Med 1996;125:257; Ann Intern Med 1997;126:946). This set point dictates the subsequent rate of progression: High concentrations (>100,000 copies/mL) are associated with a CD4 slope of -76 cells/mm^3/yr and a median survival of 4.4; low concentrations (<5000 copies/mL) are associated with a CD4 slope of -36 cells/mm^3/yr and a median survival exceeding 10 yr (Ann Intern Med 1997;126:946).

Symptomatic HIV infection.   Complications of HIV infection are ascribed to direct effects of the virus and to the consequences of immunosuppression:

- Direct effect of HIV: Acute HIV syndrome, persistent generalized lymphadenopathy (PGL), HIV-associated dementia, lymphocytic interstitial pneumonia (LIP), HIV-associated nephropathy, and progressive immunosuppression. Other possible consequences are anemia, neutropenia, thrombocytopenia, cardiomyopathy, myopathy, peripheral neuropathy, chronic meningitis, polymyositis, and Guillain-Barré syndrome.

• Immunosuppression results in opportunistic infections and tumors, primarily reflecting compromised cell-mediated immunity.

The correlation between these complications and the CD4 count as a barometer of immunocompetence is summarized in Table 5. In each instance the CD4 strata assigned is the highest in which the designated complication is likely to be encountered; virtually all conditions increase in frequency with progressive decline in CD4 count.

Early complications generally represent complications of HIV infection per se, or they are infections involving relatively virulent microbes that do not require severe immunosuppression for clinical expression. The latter include vaginal candidiasis, pneumococal pneumonia, tuberculosis, and zoster. The complications designated as AIDS-defining (Table 4) generally occur with severe immunosuppression to CD4 counts below $200/mm^3$ and usually below $100/mm^3$. The relative frequency of these complications as the original AIDS-defining diagnosis is summarized in Table 5, and their frequency as a cause of death in the pre-HAART era is summarized in Table 6.

Asymptomatic infection.   During this period the patient is asymptomatic or may have persistent generalized lymphadenopathy. There is usually a gradual decline in the CD4 cell count in untreated patients averaging $40–60/mm^3/yr$, but with substantial individual differences based on viral load and variations in the test in the test (JID 1992;165:352). The first AIDS-defining opportunistic infection occurs with an average CD4 count of $70/mm^3$ (Am J Epidemiol 1995;141:645). Note that these data on natural history are based on studies and patients who had no antiretroviral therapy or treatment with nucleosides only in the pre-HAART era. The experience with the history of HIV in patients receiving HAART is dramatically different.

Table 4. Correlation of Complications with CD4 Cell Strata

CD4 Cell Count[a]	Infections[b]	Noninfectious Complications
>500/mm³	Acute HIV syndrome *Candida* vaginitis	Persistent generalized lymphadenopathy (PGL) Polymyositis Aseptic meningitis Guillain-Barré syndrome
200–500/mm³	Pneumococcal and other bacterial pneumonia (90) Pulmonary TB (90–180) Kaposi sarcoma (30–130) Herpes zoster (150–170) Thrush Cryptosporidiosis, self-limited Oral hairy leukoplakia	Cervical intraepithelial neoplasia Cervical cancer (180) Lymphocytic interstitial pneumonitis (100–500) Mononeuronal multiplex Anemia Idiopathic thrombocytopenic purpura
<200/mm³	*P. carinii* pneumonia (40–120) *Candida* esophagitis (30–80) Disseminated/chronic Herpes simplex (40–110) Toxoplasmosis (20–40) Cryptococcosis (20–60) Disseminated histoplasmosis (30) Disseminated coccidioidomycosis (40) Cryptosporidiosis, chronic (40–130) Progressive multifocal leukoencephalopathy (PML) (40–110) Microsporidiosis (20–100) Miliary/extrapulmonary TB (40)	Wasting (20–100) B-cell lymphoma (30–60) Cardiomyopathy (25) Peripheral neuropathy (30–100) HIV-associated dementia (20–60) CNS lymphoma (20) HIV-associated nephropathy (20)
<50/mm³	CMV disease (10–20) Disseminated *M. avium* complex (10–20)	

[a] Indicated complications occur with increased frequency at lower CD4 strata; lymphomas may occur at any CD4 cell strata but are most frequent with counts <200/mm.³
[b] Number in parentheses indicates approximate median CD4 cell count at the time of diagnosis (see CID 1995;21 (Suppl 1):56; JAMA 1992;267:1798; Ann Intern Med 1996;124: 633). Some values are ranges indicating multiple sources. (CDC, MACS (A. Munoz, personal communication).)

Table 5. Frequency of Initial AIDS-Defining Diagnosis

	Initial AIDS Defining Diagnosis[a]			Frequency Among All Patients (%)[b]
	1990 (%)	1995 (%)	1997 (%)	
Pneumocystis carinii pneumonia	49	28	42	75–85
HIV wasting syndrome	17	14	11	70–90
Candida esophagitis	13	11	15	20–30
Kaposi's sarcoma	11	6	11	15–25
HIV-associated dementia	6	4	4	40–70
Disseminated CMV	6	6	4	80–90
Toxoplasmosis encephalitis	5	3	3	5–15
Disseminated *M. avium* infection	4	4	5	30–40
Lymphoma	3	2	4	3–5
Chronic mucocutaneous herpes simplex	3	4	1	10–25
Cryptococcal meningitis	3	4	—	8–12
Cryptosporidiosis	2	2	2	5–10
Tuberculosis	—	5[c]	5	4–20

[a] Frequency according to CDC criteria for AIDS 1987–1992 as reported for newly diagnosed cases in 1990 and for 1995.
[b] Estimated lifetime frequency among all patients with AIDS without prophylaxis.
[c] Added in the revised case definition of 1993.

Table 6. Causes of Death in U.S. Patients Dying of AIDS

	1987 n = 10,001	1992 n = 24,230
Pneumonia—unspecified cause	18%	18%
P. carinii pneumonia	33%	14%
Non-TB mycobacteria	7%	12%
Bacterial septicemia	9%	12%
Kaposi's sarcoma	12%	10%
CMV disease	5%	10%
Non-Hodgkin's lymphoma	4%	6%
Toxoplasmosis	5%	5%
Cryptococcosis	8%	5%
Tuberculosis	3%	4%
PML	1%	2%

4—Patient Evaluation
Summary of Guidelines of U.S. Public Health Service—Infectious Diseases Society of America (MMWR 1999; 48(RR-10); www.hivatis.org; 6/2001)

Initial Evaluation

1. Medical history. Obtain a complete medical history with emphasis on the following.
   a. *HIV serology.* Dates of positive and negative tests; necessity to confirm a positive test; reason for prior HIV test
   b. *Transmission category.* Gay male, injection drug use, heterosexual contact, transfusion, hemophilia, other or unknown
   c. *HIV-related history.* CD4 cell counts, history of AIDS-defining diagnoses
   d. *Medical care.* Usual source and care, prior PPDs, Pap smear, vaccinations (HBV, influenza, Pneumovax, tetanus HAV)
   e. *Past medical history.* Cardiovascular disease and risks for cardiovascular disease (obesity, smoking, hypertension, diabetes, family history, blood lipids). Other: Pulmonary, renal, skin, hepatic, neurologic, urologic/gynecologic, gastrointestinal, surgeries, hospitalizations
   f. *Targeted conditions relevant to HIV.* TB exposure/risk; prior chickenpox or shingles; sexually transmitted diseases; hepatitis A, B, or C; gynecologic/obstetric history; alcoholism, drug use
   g. *Medications.* For HIV, for non-HIV medical conditions, over-the-counter drugs, alternative or complementary medicine; history of compliance with HIV medications and other medications
   h. *Review of systems.* Constitutional: Weight loss, fever, night sweats, fatigue; GI: Anorexia, dysphagia, nausea, vomiting, diarrhea, abdominal pain; chest: chest pain, dyspnea, cough; neurological: headaches, weakness, painful ex-

tremeties, mental status changes, paresthesias; miscellaneous: Rashes, insomnia, adenopathy, vision

2. Patient education. Determine HIV risk behavior and assess ongoing high-risk behavior that placed patient contacts at risk. Are patients placed at risk aware of this risk? Patient education should include discussion of safe sex, safe use of needles for injection drug users, risk of childbearing, and need to test patients placed at risk. Notification of contacts will often be performed by the local health department without identification of the source, or notification may be an option offered the patient; regulations are variable in different states. All patients should be aware of the advances in HIV therapy that took place in 1996 because they revolutionized HIV care and dramatically changed outcome; they should also know that cure is unlikely with the currently available drugs.

3. Patient exam including the following:
   Oropharynx
   Lymphadenopathy
   Skin
   Heart and lungs
   Abdomen
   Genital/pelvic
   Neurologic

4. Laboratory tests
   - HIV serology (confirm prior test if necessary—should have documentation of positive serology, AIDS-defining diagnosis, or positive HIV RNA level)
   - CBC
   - CD4 count
   - Quantitative plasma HIV RNA
   - Chemistry profile including renal function and liver function tests
   - Toxoplasma serology (IgG)
   - Chest x-ray (utility of a baseline chest x-ray is questionable in patients with a negative PPD (Arch Intern Med 1996;156:191))
   - PPD (unless history of positive PPD or history of TB treatment; BCG does not preclude meaningful test results)

- STD screen; RPR or VDRL, ±GC and chlamydia urine screen (women)
- Baseline fasting lipid profile and glucose in all candidates for HAART therapy
- Hepatitis screen: Anti-HBc (to determine candidates for HBV vaccine); HBsAg and anti-HCV (to detect active hepatitis if unexplained elevated transaminase levels; anti-HCV in all injection drug users)
- Pap smear (if none in past year)
- Optional tests: CMV serology (sometimes advocated for patients in low risk categories), HAV antibody (sometimes advocated as a means to avoid unnecessary HAV vaccine in HCV co-infected patients), varicella antibody (if no history of chickenpox), G6PD (sometimes done at baseline in patients with high risk: African Americans and men of Mediterranean heritage)

5. Sequential tests

HIV RNA plasma levels: Baseline, confirmatory test at 2–4 wk, then every 3 mo if stable or more frequently with initiation of antiretroviral therapy or change in therapy

CD4 count: Baseline and then every 3–6 mo ± confirmatory test if outlier result

PPD: Annual in high-risk patients with persistently negative results

VDRL or RPR: Annual in sexually active patients

Pap smear: Baseline 6 mo, and then annually if negative

CBC: Baseline and every 3–6 mo (as a component of CD4 count)

6. Therapeutic drug monitoring

AZT—CBC every 3 mo (or more frequently)

ddC, ddI, d4T—peripheral neuropathy

Nevirapine—liver function tests, especially during first 6 wk

Protease inhibitors ± NNRTI—fasting lipid profile (cholesterol, LDL, HDL, triglycerides) at baseline and in 3–6 mo; subsequent frequency depends on risks and test results. Fasting levels necessary for triglycerides that are used to determine LDL; should be done after 8- to 12-hr fast.

7. Consultations (all are optional)

Psychiatry

Obstetrics and gynecology

Ophthalmology: Sometimes advocated for all patients with a CD4 count <100/mm^3 at 6-mo intervals

Nutrition

8. Vaccines

Pneumococcal vaccine: Recommended for patients with CD4 count >200/mm; consider in those with CD4 count <200, for those with vaccination ≥5 yr previously, and for those vaccinated with CD4 count <200 who had immune reconstitution

Influenza: Recommended; response reduced with CD4 <200/mm^3; revaccinate annually Oct–Nov

HBV vaccine: Generally recommended for those at risk with negative anti-HBVc or anti-HBVs

HAV vaccine: All patients at risk (negative anti-HAV) *and* chronic HCV infection

Tetanus booster: Should be given every 10 yr

Resources for Providers and Patients

Provider Information Resources. Resources for patient management information for providers include the following.

Guidelines of the U.S. Public Health Service and Department of Health and Human Services.

1. Antiretroviral Therapy for Adults and Adolescents: www.hivatis.org
2. Occupational Exposure: MMWR 1998;47[RR-7]
3. Prevention of Opportunistic Infections: MMWR 1999;48:RR-10
4. Antiretroviral Agents in Pregnancy: MMWR 1998;47[RR-2] Updated January 25, 2001: www.cdc.gov

AIDS education training centers. An HRSA sponsored consortium of 17 regional HIV/AIDS education centers in the U.S. to target HIV providers with emphasis on medical management; activities include a National Minority Center to facilitate access by disenfranchised patients and a National Resource Center to promote DHHS guidelines.

Websites for AIDS/HIV medical information.

www.hopkins-aids.edu

www.medscape.com

www.healtheon.com

http://hivinsite.ucsf.edu

Patient Information Resources.   Multiple information resources are available to patients that vary in content, quality, timeliness, sophistication (reading level), and language (English and Spanish primarily). The most reliable sources follow.

PWP Coalition of New York.   50 West 17th Street, New York, NY; publishes monthly "PWP Coalition Newsletter" about alternative medicines and outreach activities: 212-647-1415

Local AIDS services.   A national directory with a listing of services by geographic location from the U.S. Conference of Mayors, 1620 Eye Street, NW, Washington, DC 20006 ($15): 202-293-7330

Patient forum.   More than 2500 questions and answers in lay language available from Dr. Joel Gallant on the Johns Hopkins HIV website, which is also the recommended website for general patient education on HIV: www.hopkins-aids.edu

HIV/AIDS treatment information service.   A Public Health Service free telephone reference service for patients and providers; offers extensive library of patient information: 800-448-0440 or write PO Box 6303, Rockville, MD 20849-6303; www.hivatis.org

Therapeutic trials hotline.   National Institute of Allergy and Infectious Diseases: 1-800-TRIALS-A

American Foundation for AIDS Research (AmFar).   "AIDS/HIV Experimental Treatment Directory" (updated quarterly) and "AIDS Targeted Information Newsletter": 212-682-7440 ($125/year), www.amfar.org

Gay Men's Health Crisis (GMHC).   "Treatment Issues," GMHC, Department of Medical Information, 129 West 20th Street, New York, NY 10011: 212-807-6655 ($30/year; reliable reviews of therapeutics); Department of Education and Advocacy, 212-337-3505

National AIDS hotline.   Contracted through CDC for general information including local services: English (24 hr/day, 7 days/wk) 800-342-AIDS; Spanish (8:00 AM–2:00 PM, 7 days/wk) 1-800-344-SIDA; deaf (10:00 AM–10:00 PM, Mon–Fri) 1-800-243-7889

CDC National Prevention Information Network (HIV, STDs, TB). A library for information with publications, videos, lists of services, and community-based organizations, PO Box 6303, Rockville, MD 20849-6303: 800-458-5231

Guide to Living with HIV Infection. 2001 (4th ed), Johns Hopkins University Press, 2715 North Charles Street, Baltimore, MD 21218-4319 (paperback $15.95)

University of California at San Francisco AIDS Health Project. Psychotherapy, substance abuse counseling, HIV testing, support groups, 1855 Folsom St, Suite 670, San Francisco, CA 94103, 415-476-3902, www.ucsf-ahp.org

Bulletin of Experimental Treatments for AIDS (BETA). San Francisco AIDS Foundation; request from BETA Subscriber Services, Infocom Group, 1250 45th Street, Suite 200, Emoryville, CA 94608-2924: 800-959-1059 ($75/year; trial subscription without payment offered [suggested for the sophisticated reader])

Legal issues/civil rights. Office of Civil Rights, Department of Health and Human Services, PO Box 13716, Mail Stop 07, Philadelphia, PA 19101: 215-596-6109; social security—disability qualifications: 800-772-1213

National Institute on Drug Abuse hotline. Substance abuse referral and printed material resource: English 800-662-4357; Spanish 800-662-9832

Project Inform. HIV treatment information, treatment hotline and advocacy with publications and services. 1-800-822-7422, www.projinf.org

National Association of People with AIDS. NAPWA 1413 K St NW, 7th floor Wash DC 20005 www.napwa.org 202-898-0414. Information about local resources, including support groups, mail order pharmacy, update information on new treatments, and two quarterly publications: "Medical Alert" (treatments) and "Active Voice" (advocacy)

"Wellness": Exercise, Smoking, Alcohol. Medical care should include appropriate attention to nutrition, exercise, continued work, and other facets of "wellness." Depression does not appear to accelerate disease progression (JAMA 1993;270: 2563). Three separate studies have demonstrated deleterious consequences of smoking with increased rates of PCP and more rapid progression to AIDS (AIDS 1990;4:327). It is unknown if effective PCP prophylaxis would nullify the disadvantage.

Strenuous exercise as done by Olympic athletes or marathon runners is deleterious to immune function with increased susceptibility to common viral infections but is not known to reduce cell-mediated immunity; moderate exercise such as jogging or bicycle riding has no apparent adverse effect on immune function and may improve sense of well-being. Alcohol in moderation (one drink per day) has no adverse health consequences including problems with immune function, infections, rates of liver disease, or rates of hepatotoxicity with AZT, INH, etc; obviously, alcohol may reduce inhibitions and enhance high-risk behavior and also promote side effects of psychiatric or sedative drugs. Of particular concern is the effect alcohol has on compliance with complex medical regimens, especially binge drinking. HIV and alcohol are the two-way co-factors adding risk of progression with HCV; HIV-infected patients with HCV co-infection should not drink alcohol at all. Nutrition needs emphasis, but it is unknown whether routine nutrition consults, specific diets, vitamin supplements, or mineral supplements are advantageous (Lancet 1991;338:86; Nutr Rev 1990;48:393). Unusual diets such as macrobiotic diet and megavitamins may be dangerous.

Role of Pets, Food, Travel, and Occupational Risks
(Ann Intern Med 1997;127:939)

Pets.   The major concern with pets is that they may carry the microbes that cause diarrhea in patients, primarily *Cryptosporidia, Salmonella,* and *Campylobacter.* The following precautions will help avoid this type of exposure and are relevant primarily to those with a CD4 count $<200/\text{mm}^3$: Veterinary consultation should be obtained if the pet develops diarrhea. When obtaining a new pet, avoid animals younger than 6 mo, pets with diarrhea, stray animals, and animals from facilities that have poor hygienic conditions. Wash hands after handling pets and especially before eating, and avoid contact with stool. If a pet develops diarrhea, it should be examined by a veterinarian.

Cats are of particular concern owing to risk of exposure to toxoplasmosis and *Bartonella,* as well as the microbes that cause diarrhea. It is best to obtain a cat older than 1 yr that is in good health. Litter boxes should be cleaned daily, preferably by someone who is not infected with HIV nor is pregnant. If this must be done by an HIV-infected person, hands should be washed thoroughly afterward to reduce the risk. Cats should be kept indoors, should not hunt, and should not be fed raw or undercooked meat because all of these increase the risk of toxoplasmosis. *Bartonella* is transmitted by bites and scratches of cats, and these should be avoided and should be cleaned promptly when they occur. It is not suggested to declaw a cat or test the animal for either toxoplasmosis or *Bartonella* infection.

With regard to other pets, healthy birds may be the source of cryptococcus or *Histoplasma*. Reptiles such as snakes and turtles may carry *Salmonella*. Aquariums are generally safe, but gloves should be used for cleaning to reduce exposure to *Mycobacterium marinum*. Nonhuman primates like monkeys should be avoided.

Food.   The major risk with food and fluids is exposure to the microbes that cause diarrhea. Most enteric pathogens cause diarrhea in any host after exposure. The two that are particularly problematic to patients with AIDS are cryptosporidiosis, which can cause debilitating and chronic diarrhea in those with a CD4 count of $<180/mm^3$ and *Salmonella*, which commonly causes bacteremia in AIDS. *Salmonella* is often present in eggs and poultry, and undercooked meat is a common source of toxoplasmosis. The usual recommendation is to avoid raw or undercooked eggs, including the foods that often contain raw eggs such as hollandaise sauce and Caesar salad dressing. Also avoid raw or undercooked poultry, seafood, and meat. Poultry and meat should be cooked until it is no longer pink in the middle. Produce should be washed thoroughly before it is eaten. Patients should be reminded of the possibility of exposure to undercooked meats or other products through contact with cutting boards, counters, knives, and hands used in preparation; all should be washed carefully.

Warn patients to not drink directly from lakes or rivers because of the risk of cryptosporidiosis. There are sometimes community outbreaks of diarrhea in which there is a "boil-water" advisory. At such a time the water should be boiled 1 min to remove the risk of *Cryptosporidium* and other disease-causing microbes. Other options are submicron personal-use water filters and/or bottled water. The submicron filter recommended is one that is labeled "absolute" 1-μm filter; the best are those labeled to show they meet National Sanitation Foundation Standard number 53 for "cyst removal." Note that many filters labeled 1 μm are not standardized and are consequently not recommended. It is not generally recommended that HIV-infected persons boil the water or use tap water filtration if there is no advisory, but some may choose to use these precautions to be extra cautious.

Travel   (CID 2000;31:1403). The greatest health risk to persons with and without HIV infection is visits to developing countries, and the major problem is microbes that contaminate food and water. Avoid raw fruits and vegetables, raw or undercooked seafood or meat, tap water, ice made from tap water, nonpasteurized milk and dairy products, and items purchased from street vendors. The preferred foods are those that are steaming hot, fruits that can be peeled by the traveler, bottled water, hot coffee or tea, or anything with alcohol in it. Water may also be treated with iodine or chlorine, but this is not as effective as a rolling boil for 1 min. These recommendations apply to all travelers regardless of HIV status (CID 2000;32:331).

Antibiotics to prevent infections during travel to developing countries are usually not recommended, but they may be for some HIV-infected patients who are considered at high risk. A common recommendation is for a fluoroquinolone to prevent or treat diarrhea. Trimethoprim-sulfamethoxazole (TMP-SMX) is sometimes used, which many travelers may already be taking to prevent *Pneumocystis* pneumonia. It is important to be aware of the side effects of TMP-SMX when taken for prophylaxis during travel because these may appear to be some tropical disease. The most common reaction is a rash and fever, and the only treatment necessary is to simply stop the drug. For travelers to developing countries who do not take antibiotics, it is generally recommended to take loperamide for the treatment of mild diarrhea ($\leq$2 loose stools/24 hr) or loperamide plus a fluoroquinolone for more severe diarrhea or diarrhea associated with fever and constitutional symptoms. The standard dose of loperamide is 4 mg, then 2 mg with each loose stool for a maximum of 16 mg/d. The dose of ciprofloxacin is 500 mg bid $\times$ 1–3 days; other fluoroquinolones are probably equally effective, especially ofloxacin, levofloxacin, or norfloxacin.

Vaccines are often required or recommended for travel, and

Table 7. Vaccines for Travel

Disease	Acceptable	Avoid	Comment
Polio	eIPV	Oral polio	Close contacts should also receive eIPV
Hepatitis A	—	HAV vaccine	Live virus vaccine; use gammaglobulin
Typhoid	Typhim Vi	Ty21a (Vivotif)	Inactivated parenteral vaccine is also acceptable
Jap B encephalitis	JBE vaccine	—	
Yellow fever	—	Vaccine—avoid with CD4 < 200	Advise patient of risk and risk prevention (mosquito) and provide waiver
Meningitis	Meningo-cocceal vaccine	—	Use when indicated by travel to meningitis belt of Africa or when indicated by outbreaks

recommendations are made in Table 7. The general rule is that HIV-infected persons cannot receive live virus vaccines. If there is anticipated exposure to typhoid fever, the inactivated injected vaccine is recommended rather than the live vaccine form that is given by mouth. For yellow fever, the only vaccine is a live virus vaccine that has uncertain safety in people with HIV infection; if there is travel to an area with yellow fever, it may be necessary to obtain a letter indicating vaccination waiver, and there must be extra caution in avoiding mosquito bites. Killed vaccines are not a problem; these include the standard diphtheria-tetanus, rabies, meningococcal vaccines, and Japanese encephalitis vaccines.

Travelers must be aware about the types of infectious diseases that may pose particular risks in various areas. When malaria prophylaxis is indicated, there is concern about drug interactions between mefloquin and protease inhibitors. Preferred alternative for the patient taking HAART are doxycycline, chloroquin, atovaquones and proquainil. Many developing countries have high rates of tuberculosis, and HIV-infected persons are more than 100 times more likely to get this infection than persons without HIV infection. Many areas pose a risk for malaria, and the standard precautions include avoidance of insect bites and certain preventive drugs that should not be a problem for HIV-infected persons. Visceral leishmaniasis (kala azar) is a disease transmitted by sandflies in many tropical countries that can be a major problem in patients with HIV infection. This includes South and Central America (New World) and Asia, Africa, and Southern Europe (Old World). The same applies to *Penicillium marneffei* in the Far East: Thailand, Hong Kong, China, Vietnam, Indonesia (Lancet 1994;344:110).

Despite these concerns, there is relatively little to support the claim that travel, even in late stages of HIV infection, is too dangerous owing to exposures in other countries if simple precautions are taken.

Occupational Risks.   The major occupational risks to persons with HIV infection are in health care and child care and occupations that require animal contact. In the health care field, the major risk is tuberculosis exposure; this might also apply to employment in correctional facilities, shelters for the homeless, and volunteers for these sites. The specific risk depends to a large extent on the activities of the worker/volunteer and the prevalence of tuberculosis in the community. The major risk to providers of child care are *Cryptosporidium* and, to a lesser extent, *Cytomegalovirus,* hepatitis A, and giardiasis. The risk may be substantially reduced simply by good hygiene. Occupations requiring animal contact include veterinary work and employment in farms, slaughterhouses, or pet stores. The major risks are for *Cryptosporidium, Toxoplasma, Salmonella, Campylobacter,* and *Bartonella.* There is not good evidence that these occupations are sufficiently risky to avoid continued employment; the recommendation is to be aware of the risk and use appropriate precautions.

Most Common Presentations

Major diagnostic considerations based on physical findings are summarized in Table 8.

Laboratory Testing

The usual laboratory tests performed with initial evaluation are designed to (*a*) ensure confirmation of HIV infection; (*b*) stage the disease; (*c*) identify latent pathogens that will influence subsequent strategies for treatment and prophylaxis; and (d) determine general health status. Specific guidelines are summarized in Table 9.

HIV Serology. Guidelines for HIV serology in terms of indications, interpretation, and use of alternative tests are summarized in Chapter 1. The test should be repeated for confirmation if there is no report of a prior positive test or no confirmation as with CD4 count, AIDS-defining complicating viral load etc. CD4 counts may serve as a surrogate marker for advanced HIV infection in patients with possible HIV-related complications when serology results are delayed or serology is refused. The CBC can be used to detect lymphopenia ($<1000/mm^3$), which is supportive. A CD4 count is more specific because relatively few conditions in medicine other than HIV cause severe depletion of CD4 cells; acute corticosteroid therapy may cause this. HIV serology is clearly more sensitive and specific, although there are relatively few medical conditions associated with counts of $<300/mm^3$ (NEJM 1993;328:373,380,386,393).

CD4 Cell Count. Mean levels in healthy controls for most laboratories are $800–1050/mm^3$, with a range representing two standard deviations of about $450–1400/mm^3$ (Ann Intern Med 1993;119:55). There is substantial variation in the test results owing to technology, diurnal variations, and possible influence of intercurrent illnesses. Diurnal variations show lowest levels at 12:30 PM and peak values at 8:30 PM. The average diurnal change in HIV-infected persons with counts of 200–500 is $60/mm^3$ (J AIDS 1990;3:144). Marked laboratory variations reflect the fact that the count represents the product of three variables: White blood cell count, percent lymphocytes, and percent lymphocytes that bear the CD4 receptor. High-quality laboratories participating in ACTG trials showed the average within-subject coefficient of variation was 25% (JID 1994;169:28). A comparison of four labs performing tests on 24 patients showed the average difference between high and low values was $108/mm^3$; 14 of the 24 had results that would lead to different therapeutic decisions (CID 1995;21:1121). The 95% confidence limits indicate that the reporting range for a value of $500/mm^3$ is $297–841/mm^3$. Standards for quality assurance have recently been published by the CDC (MMWR 1997;46(RR-2)). Methods to reduce variations are to use the same laboratory, sample patients at times of clinical

Table 8. Major Diagnostic Considerations by Organ System[a]

Conditions	CD4 >300/mm^3	CD4 <200/mm^3
Lymphadenopathy	PGL (syphilis, lymphoma, KS, TB)	PGL (CMV, TB, KS, MA)
Eye (fundi)		
Exudate + hemorrhage	HIV retinopathy	CMV retinitis
Cotton wool spots		HIV retinopathy
Oral		
White patches	Thrush, OHL	Thrush, OHL
Ulcers	HSV, aphthous ulcers	HSV, aphthous ulcers, CMV
Red-purple nodular lesions	KS	KS
Esophagus (dysphagia)		*Candida*, CMV, aphthous ulcers (HSV)
Abdomen		
Diarrhea	*Salmonella, C. difficile, Campylobacter, Shigella,* viral agents, cryptosporidiosis	*Cryptosporidium*, microsporidia, MA, CMV, adverse drug reaction, *C. difficile*, AIDS enteropathy (small bowel overgrowth, histoplasmosis, isospora, cyclospora, lymphoma)
Hepatomegaly and/or abnormal LFTs	Hepatitis (usually HBV or HCV), adverse drug reaction	Hepatitis (HBV or HCV), CMV, MA, lactic acidosis, lymphoma, HIV, fatty liver secondary to malnutrition; cholangiopathy-*Cryptosporidium*, CMV, idiopathic, (microsporidia)
Splenomegaly	HIV	Lymphoma, MA, histoplasmosis, HIV, cirrhosis

Skin

Purple-black nodular lesions	KS (bacillary angiomatosis, prurigo nodularis)
Vesicles	Herpes simplex, herpes zoster
Maculopapular lesions	Adverse drug reaction, syphilis
Plaques, scaling lesions	Seborrhea (psoriasis, eczema)
Umbilicated papules	Molluscum
Petechiae, purpura	ITP
Nodules	Cryptococcus, histoplasmosis, pruritis nodularis

Lungs

| Pneumonia | S. pneumoniae, (H. influenzae, TB, aspiration, atypical agents) |
| Cavity, nodules | TB (S. aureus with IV drug users) |

Neurological

Aseptic meningitis	Neurosyphilis, viral
Chronic meningitis	Tuberculosis, neurosyphilis
Dementia	Trauma, tumor, depression, hypothyroid

Constitutional symptoms
(FUO, weight loss, etc)

| | Lymphoma, TB |

KS (bacillary angiomatosis, prurigo nodularis)
Herpes simplex, herpes zoster (CMV)
Adverse drug reaction, syphilis
Seborrhea (psoriasis, eczema)
Molluscum (cryptococcus)
ITP
Cryptococcus, histoplasmosis, pruritis nodularis

PCP, bacterial infections (TB, MA, KS, CMV, cryptococcus, histoplasmosis, lymphocytic interstitial pneumonia)
TB (cryptococcus, nocardia, KS, lymphoma, MA, M. kansasii, atypical PCP, Rhodococcus, Aspergillus)

Cryptococcus
Cryptococcus, tuberculosis, neurosyphilis
HIV-associated dementia

MA, CMV, histoplasmosis, HIV, cryptococcosis, PCP, lymphoma

---

[a] CMV, cytomegalovirus; PCP, P. carinii pneumonia; MA, M. avium; TB, tuberculosis; OHL, oral hairy leukoplakia; PGL, peripheral generalized lymphadenopathy; HSV, herpes simplex virus; ADC, AIDS dementia complex.
[b] Conditions in parentheses indicate less likely diagnoses.

Table 9. Routine Laboratory Tests in Patients with HIV Infection (see DHHS Guidelines: MMWR 1998;47(RR-3):38)

Test	Cost	Frequency	Comment
HIV serology	Average $40	Once	• Repeat test for patients who have no identified risks, no confirmed test if plasma HIV RNA is negative or not done
CBC	$6–8	Every 3–6 mo	• Repeat more frequently with marrow suppression
CD4 count	$40–150	Every 3–6 mo	• Standard method to monitor immunocompetency • Routine testing is unnecessary for untreated patients with CD4 count <50/mm³ • Outlier results should be confirmed owing to large variations in test results
Plasma HIV RNA	$80–240	Every 3–4 mo and 4–8 wk after new therapy	• Standard method to evaluate prognosis and response to therapy • Recommendation is baseline tests × 2 separated by ≥2 wk; with initiation of treatment or change in treatment. Test should be repeated at 4–8 wk to determine initial response (alpha slope) and at 4–6 mo to determine maximal effect (beta slope) • Testing should be done using same lab, same technique, at a time of clinical stability, and ≥1 mo from immunizations
Serum chemistries	$10–15	Annual or more frequent	• Major interest is hepatic function test owing to high rates of chronic hepatitis • Monitoring more frequently is necessary with use of nephrotoxic or hepatotoxic drugs including NNRTIs and PIs
Anti-HBc	$10–15	Once in candidates for HBV vaccine	• Candidate for HBV vaccine

Test	Cost	Frequency	Comments
Anti-HCV and HBsAg	$40–60	Once in patient with unexplained abnormal LFTs	
Toxoplasma IgG	$12–15	Once (see comments)	• Screen all patients and repeat in seronegatives if 1) CD4 count <100/mm^3 and patient does not take TMP-SMX prophylaxis and 2) symptoms suggesting toxoplasmosis
PPD	$1	Annually	• Indicated if no history of positive PPD or treatment of TB • Repeat annually if high risk of TB and with exposure
Chest x-ray	$40–100	See comment	• Commonly advocated at baseline but prior study of 1065 HIV-infected patients showed virtually no useful information (Arch Intern Med 1996;156:191) • Indicated in patients with positive PPD, history of chest disease, or pulmonary symptoms
PAP smear	$25–40	Baseline, 6 mo, then annually	• Repeat results reported as inadequate • Refer to gynecologist for atypia or greater on the Bethesda score
CMV serology	$10–15	See comment	• Advocated for detection of latent CMV in low-risk patients to 1) permit counseling for CMV prevention (same as HIV), 2) assist in differential diagnosis of possible CMV disease, and 3) guide use of CMV-antibody negative blood or leukocyte-reduced blood products
VDRL or RPR	$5–16	Annually in sexually active patients	• Positives must have FTA confirmation: Up to 6% of HIV-infected patients have false-positive screening tests (CID 1994;19:1040; Am J Med 1995;99:55)
Fasting lipid profile and glucose		Baseline and at 3–6 mo in patients given PIs	• Purpose is to evaluate risk for atherosclerosis and diabetes as complications of treatment with protease inhibitors and possibly with NNRTIs • Frequency of testing during therapy depends on results at 3–6 mo and additional risks

stability, and maintain consistency in the time of blood draws. Some clinicians prefer the CD4 percent because this reduces variation to one measurement (J AIDS 1989;2:114). Corresponding CD4 cell counts follow:

CD4 Cell Count	%CD4
>500/mm^3	>29
200–500/mm^3	14–28
<200/mm^3	<14

Medical conditions that cause modest decreases in CD4 cell count include acute CMV infection, hepatitis B infection, tuberculosis, some bacterial infections, and major surgery. Corticosteroid administration may have a profound effect with decreases from 900 to <300/mm^3 after acute administration of high doses; chronic administration has a much less pronounced effect. Strenuous exercise may lower absolute lymphocyte subsets (MMWR 1997;46:1). Coinfection with HTLV-1 and splenectomy may be responsible for a deceptively high CD4 count. Factors that have minimal effect are gender, age in adults, risk category, psychological stress, physical stress, and pregnancy (Ann Intern Med 1993;119:55).

Quantitative HIV RNA.   Plasma HIV RNA level measurement (viral load) is a standard method to evaluate patients with HIV and to measure response to therapy. The best data for its prognostic value are from the Multicenter AIDS Cohort Study (MACS), which is a prospective longitudinal study of HIV infection in gay men that was initiated in 1984. Frozen sera from this cohort were analyzed for correlation with clinical outcome according to assessments at 6-mo intervals for the ensuing decade; results are summarized in Table 10 (Ann Intern Med 1997; 126:946). Multiple subsequent reports have confirmed the clinical utility of VL testing for determining prognosis and for therapeutic monitoring. The MACS data show that VL is a strong predictor of progression that is independent of the CD4. The goal of therapy is "no detectable virus." Initial tests had a threshold of detection of 400–500 copies/mL; "second generation tests" or "ultrasensitive tests" then had a threshold of 20–50

Table 10. Quantitative HIV RNA

	Roche* 800-526-1247	Bayer (Formerly Chiron) 800-434-2447	Organon 800-682-2666 × 152
Technique	RT-PCR	bDNA	NASBA
Dynamic range	Amplicor HIV-1 1.0: 400–750,000 copies/mL Ultrasensitive: 40–75,000 copies/mL	Version 3.0 (preferred): 100–500,000 copies/mL Version 2.0: 500–500,000 copies/mL	Nuclisens HIV-1 QT: 40–10,000,000 copies/mL depending on volume
Subtypes quantitated	Version 1.0-B Version 1.5-A–G	A–G	A–F (G)
Specimen volume	Amplicor 1.0: 0.2 mL Ultrasensitive: 0.5 mL	1 mL	10 µL–2 mL
Tubes	EDTA (lavender top)	EDTA (lavender top)	EDTA, heparin, whole blood, body fluid, semen, tissue, etc
Relative merits	Amplicor 1.0 is only one that is FDA approved Amplicor 1.0 quantitate only subtype B; other subtypes are low. Version 1.5 quantitates subgroups A–G	Technician demand is less Quantitates subtypes A–G	Will quantitate HIV in many body fluids and tissue Quantitates subtypes A–G

* Amplicor version 1.0 is to be phased out.

Table 11. Viral Burden Analysis

Viral Burden (copies/mL)*	No. of Patients	Relative Hazard		Median Survival (yr)	CD4 Slope
		AIDS	Death		
<500	112	1.0	1.0	>10	−36
500–3,000	229	2.4	2.8	>10	−45
3,000–10,000	347	4.4	5.0	>10	−55
10,000–30,000	357	7.6	9.9	7.5	−65
>30,000	386	13	18.5	4.4	−76

* MACS data (Ann Intern Med 1997;126:946).

copies/mL; it is expected that commercially available tests in the future will detect 2–5 copies/mL.

There are three commercially available methods to measure viral load that are summarized in Table 11. The reproducibility of these tests is about 0.3 $\log_{10}$ copies/mL or about 2-fold. Results with RT-PCR are twice the levels with bDNA (J Clin Microbiol 2000;38:2837); comparative values for the Nuclisens assay are not available. Plasma HIV RNA levels in early stage HIV are about 2-fold lower in women compared with men for the same prognosis in terms of CD4 count, AIDS defining complications, or death; these differences disappear with progression to later stages (Lancet 1998;352:1510; NEJM 2001;344:720).

Resistance Testing.   This is an in vitro method to measure susceptibility of HIV strains to antiretroviral agents. There are two basic methods that have different merits.

Genotypic assays.   Genotypic assays measure mutations on the reverse transcriptase (RT) or protease (P) gene. Mutations are reported for each gene using a letter-number-letter standard in which the first letter indicates the amino acid at the designated codon in wild-type virus; the number is the codon, and the second letter indicates the substituted amino acid (Table 12) (J AIDS 23:53, 2001). Resistance mutations are classified as "primary" or "secondary" for protease inhibitors. This distinction has been discontinued for mutations on the RT gene.

Phenotypic assays.   Phenotypic assays are offered by Virco and ViroLogic. These are more analogous to conventional antibacterial sensitivity tests with results reported as the -fold in-

Table 12. Codon Mutations that Confer Resistance to Antiretroviral Agents
(Updates Available at http://hiv-web.lanl.gov)*

Protease Gene	Primary	Secondary
Indinavir	46, 82	10, 20, 24, 46, 63, 64, 82, 84, 90
Ritonavir	82	8, 10, 20, 33, 36, 46, 54, 63, 71, 84, 90
Saquinavir	48, 90	10, 24, 30, 46, 54, 63, 64, 71, 73, 77, 81, 84, 88
Nelfinavir	30, 90	10, 35, 36, 46, 71, 88
Amprenavir	50, 84	10, 32, 46, 47, 50, 54
Lopinavir	—	10, 20, 24, 46, 53, 63, 71, 82, 84, 90

RT Gene		
Zidovudine	41, 67, 70, 210, 215, 219	
Didanosine	65, 74, 184	
Zalcitabine	65, 69, 184	
Lamivudine	184, —	
Stavudine	75	
Abacavir	41, 65, 67, 70, 74, 115, 184, 210, 215, 219	
Multiple NRTI	41, 62, 67, 69, 70, 75, 77, 116, insertion 151 210, 215, 219	
Nevirapine	100, 103, 106, 108, 181, 188, 190, 230	
Efavirenz	100, 103, 108, 188, 190, 225, 230	
Delavirdine	103, 181, 230, 236	

* JAMA 2000;283:2417.

crease in resistance compared with wild-type virus. The levels selected to define resistance were formerly quite arbitrary, usually 1.7-, 4-, or 10-fold higher than wild-type virus, meaning the test strain was 1.7-, 4-, or 10-fold more resistant than wild-type virus for any specific drug. The present reporting system uses different thresholds for each drug based on clinical trial experience and other data (JID 2001;183:401). PI combinations with RTV booster are problematic.

Virtual phenotype.   This is a combination of both methods using the genotypic assay to define mutations, which is then matched with the phenotype of previously tested strains that have the same mutational pattern.

Relative merits of assays.   There are two limitations for both types of assays. 1) They measure only the dominant HIV species; variants that account for <20% of the total viral population tested are not tested. The implication is that resistant

Table 13. Comparison of Genotypic and Phenotypic Assays to Detect HIV Resistance

	Genotypic Assay	Phenotypic Assay
Availability	Widely available	Less readily available
Cost	$360–$480/test for RT and P gene	$800–$1000
Turnaround time	7–14 days	14–21 days
Viral load required	>1000 copies/mL	>1000 copies/mL
Interpretation	Requires knowledge of effect of each mutational change	More analogous to in vitro sensitivity tests for bacteria, but there are uncertain definitions of thresholds that indicate clinically significant resistance
	Results are confounded by incomplete knowledge of resistance mutations	
	May fail to correlate with phenotypic resistance	Measures total effect
	Very reproducible	Very reproducible
		Two suppliers (ViroLogic and Virco): Both validated and never compared

strains may not be detected so that results are most accurate in defining drugs that will not be effective rather than those that will work. Samples for testing should be obtained while patients are receiving failed therapy to promote testing of agents in the current regimen. 2) Neither assay can be performed on specimens with viral loads <1000 copies/mL. 3) A third limitation is the difficulty in interpreting results with both assays. Relative merits of the tests are summarized in Table 13 (J AIDS 2001;26: 53).

Indications. Resistance testing is advocated according to the DHHS guidelines (www.hivatis.org).

Recommendations. Virologic failure—select the next regimen and preserve options. This is the only category in which there is a demonstrated benefit of resistance testing compared with "standard care" (physician decision based on historical information about drug exposures). Resistance testing may be used to facilitate therapeutic decisions with suboptimal response at 8–16 wk or with failure to achieve complete viral suppression at 16–24 wk or later.

Considerations.   Resistance testing in acute HIV syndrome may allow optimal drug selection (BMJ 2001;322:1087).

No recommendations.   Initial treatment of chronically infected patients because wild-type virus usually dominates in untreated chronically infected patients despite the possible presence of resistant strains that then emerge with antiretroviral therapy. Patients off therapy should not be tested; about 2–6 wk is required for emergence of the deceptively susceptible wild-type virus. Patients with a viral load of <1000 copies/mL should not be tested because the test cannot be reliably performed on this population.

Syphilis Serology.   Screening tests (VDRL or RPR) should be performed with the initial evaluation and repeated annually in patients who are sexually active. False-negative and false-positive tests have been reported in patients with HIV infection (JID 1990;162:862; JID 1992;165:1020; AIDS 1991;5:419), but these are rare (Ann Intern Med 1990;113:872). Patients with a positive screening test should have a confirmatory fluorescent treponemal antibody absorption test.

Serum Chemistry Panel.   The screen should include tests of liver function (bilirubin, transaminase levels, alkaline phosphatase), renal function, and glucose.

Hepatitis B Serology.   HBsAg is tested to determine if the patient has chronic hepatitis caused by HBV; many such patients are candidates for therapy with interferon or lamivudine. Anti-HBc is measured to determine candidates for HBV vaccine. Patients with HIV have a CD4 cell count dependent response—only 50–70% with low CD4 counts develop antibody levels of >10 units/mL after three doses; these patients are candidates for one additional three dose series.

Hepatitis C.   About 90% of injection drug users have positive HCV serology, and about 85% of men are chronic carriers (MMWR 1998;47(RR-19)). Indications for anti-HCV include injection drug use and unexplained abnormal liver function tests. The only FDA-approved screening test is anti-HCV, which has a 97% sensitivity for chronic HCV infection but has a low predictive value (specificity) in low prevalence populations and fails to distinguish acute, chronic, and resolved infection (Hepatology 1997;26:435). Positive anti-HCV screening tests should be supplemented with RT-PCR for HCV RNA to confirm the diagnosis. Quantitative HCV RNA is positive in 75–85% of persons with anti-HCV tests and >95% of patients with acute or chronic HCV infection. Tests that will identify patients with chronic HCV infection who are candidates for therapy are HCV RNA levels (RT-PCR or bDNA), ALT, liver biopsy, and genotypic assays. Genotype 1 accounts for 70% of chronic HCV infections, which respond poorly to therapy. The algorithm is EIA for anti-HCV screening → if positive RT-PCR for HCV RNA → if either is positive → medical evaluation for therapy and prognosis: ALT, quantitative HCV RNA, liver biopsy, and genotypic assay of HCV.

Toxoplasmosis Serology.   IgG for *T. gondii* is advocated 1) at the initial screen to determine latent infection, 2) in previously seronegative or untested patients who become candidates for toxoplasmosis prophylaxis using agents other than TMP-SMX (given for PCP prophylaxis) because of a CD4 count of <100/mm^3, and 3) in previously seronegative or untested patients who have possible CNS toxoplasmosis. Seroprevalence for adults in the U.S. is usually 10–30%; sensitivity of the test in patients with CNS toxoplasmosis is 90–100%.

Cytomegalovirus Serology.   This is sometimes advocated with initial evaluation to detect latent CMV infection in patients with a low risk of harboring CMV. Seroprevalence of CMV in healthy adults in the U.S. is 50–70%; it is >90% in gay men, IDUs, and hemophiliacs.

PPD Skin Test.   The CDC recommends routine testing with PPD (using the standard Mantoux test) 5TU units with interpretation at 48–72 hr by a health care professional. A prospective study of 1130 HIV-infected persons followed a median of 53 mo showed the rate of active TB was 0.5/100 in those who remained PPD negative compared with 3.2/100 in those with baseline positive PPD tests and 4.7/100 in those who seroconverted (Ann Intern Med 1997;126:123). There is consensus that the PPD test should have a high priority, but anergy testing is no longer recommended because of lack of standard-

Table 14. Management of Abnormal Pap Smear Test Results: Recommendations of the Agency for Health Care Policy and Research and National Cancer Institute

Results	Action
Inadequate	Repeat
Inflammation	Evaluate for infection, treat, and repeat Pap smear in 2–3 mo
Atypia (ASCUS)	Repeat Pap smear every 4–6 mo × 2 yr to achieve three consecutive negative smears or colposcopy
Low-grade squamous intraepithelial lesion (LGSIL or LSIL) (CIN 1)	Colcoposcopy and biopsy or follow-up Pap smear every 4–6 mo; consider repeat colcoposcopy annually
High-grade squamous intraepithelial lesions (HGSIL or HSIL) (CIN 2 or 3)	Colposcopy and biopsy; treat with loop excision or conization
Invasive carcinoma	Refer to gynecologic oncologist for surgery or radiation

From JAMA 1994;271:1866.

ization of reagents and inconsistent results with repeat tests in HIV-infected patients (Arch Intern Med 1993;155:2111). The definition of a positive PPD in HIV-infected patients is ≥5 mm induration.

Pap Smear.   The CDC recommends a gynecologic evaluation with pelvic examination and Pap smear in women with HIV infection at initial evaluation, a repeat Pap smear 6 mo later, and then annually if results are normal (MMWR 1990;39:47). Current recommendations for managing results are shown in Table 14.

Chest X-Ray.   A chest x-ray is recommended for detection of asymptomatic TB and also as a baseline test for patients who have high rates of pulmonary disease. A review of screening chest x-rays in 1065 HIV-infected persons at 0-, 3-, 6-, and 12-mo intervals showed only 2% were abnormal, and this technique detected only 11 of 55 patients who developed pulmonary complications within 2 mo of the x-ray. The yield was also low in groups at high risk for TB and those with low CD4 counts. The authors concluded that chest x-rays as a screening test in asymptomatic HIV-infected persons with a negative PPD are unwarranted (Arch Intern Med 1996;156:191).

Lipid Profile.   Patients who are candidates for HAART should have a baseline analysis of cholesterol (HDL and LDL), fasting triglycerides, and fasting blood glucose. This should be repeated about 3–6 mo after initiating a regimen containing a protease inhibitor or an NNRTI. Most patients who have blood lipid abnormalities or insulin resistance will show abnormal test results within 3–4 mo. These results become the database for decisions regarding changes in treatment or introduction of methods to prevent atheroscelerosis using the National Cholesterol Education guidelines (see Table 34). The frequency of testing in patients who have normal tests at 3–4 mo is not well defined. Abnormal blood glucose levels should be managed according to guidelines for diabetic control.

Glucose-6-Phosphate Dehydrogenase Level.   Glucose-6-phosphate dehydrogenase (G-6-PD) deficiency is a genetic disease that predisposes to hemolytic anemia after exposure to oxidant drugs. There are more than 300 variants that are inherited on the X chromosome. The most common form is GdA, which is found in 10% of black males and 1–2% of black females; the most serious form is GdMED, which is found predominantly in males from the Mediterranean area (Italians, Greeks, Sephardic Jews, Arabs) and males from India and Southeast Asia. In most cases, the hemolysis is mild and self-limited because only the older red cells are involved and the bone marrow can compensate. The most important exception is GdMED, which may cause life-threatening hemolysis. The severity of anemia also depends on concentration of the drug in the red cells and the oxidant potential; the most likely offending agents used in patients with HIV infection are dapsone and primaquine and less likely are sulfonamides. During hemolysis, G-6-PD levels are usually normal because the susceptible red cells have been destroyed so that testing must be delayed for about 1 mo after a drug holiday. Methemoglobin levels will be elevated. Options for testing are to 1) obtain this test at baseline; 2) screen patients at high risk (African-American males and males of Mediterranean descent); 3) delay testing until oxidant drugs are indicated; or

4) delay until hemolysis is suspected (with measurement of methemoglobin acutely and level of G-6-PD after a drug holiday). Most patients with low levels tolerate oxidant drugs well; it would be a mistake to consider, for example, TMP-SMX or dapsone to be absolutely contraindicated in an African-American male with an abnormally low G-6-PD level.

5—Prevention: Opportunistic Infections
USPHS/IDSA Guidelines (MMWR 1999; 48(RR-10))

The U.S. Public Health Service and the Infectious Diseases Society of America provided guidelines on strategies to reduce the frequency of opportunistic infections that were originally published in 1995 (MMWR 1995;44(RR-8); CID 1995;21(Suppl 1)) and revised in 1997 (Ann Intern Med 1997;127:939). Revised recommendations are presented in the following tables.

Table 15: Prevention of Opportunistic Infections: Antimicrobial Prophylaxis

Table 16: Recommendations for Primary and Secondary Opportunistic Infection Prophylaxis during Pregnancy

Table 17: Recommendations for Vaccines in HIV-Infected Patients

Table 15. Prevention of Opportunistic Infections: Antimicrobial Prophylaxis
Recommendation of USPHS/IDSA (MMWR 1999;48(RR-10))

Disease	Indications: Start and Stop*	Preferred Regimen (cost/mo)	Comment/Alternative/Stopping recs (www.hivatis.org 8/01)
STRONGLY RECOMMENDED AS STANDARD OF CARE			
Tuberculosis (latent)	PPD + (≥5 mm induration) Prior positive PPD without prior INH prophylaxis High-risk exposure	INH 300 mg/d + pyridoxine 50 mg/d ≥270 doses, 9 mo or up to 12 mo with interruptions ($2.00/mo) INH 900 mg + pyridoxine 100 mg 2×/wk with DOT ≥76 doses, 9 mo or up to 12 mo with interruptions ($0.60/mo)	Rifampin 600 mg/d + pyrazinamide 20 mg/kg/d with ≥60 doses × 2 mo or up to 3 mo with interruptions ($268/mo) • Alternative (INH resistance or toxicity): Rifampin 600 mg/d × 4 mo • Alternative for patient receiving PI or NNRTI who needs substitute for rifampin. Give rifabutin, pyrazinamide 20 mg/kg/d × 2 mo, and modified PI/NNRTI dose PI or NNRTI Rifabutin APV—standard + RBT 150 mg/d or 300 mg 2×/wk IDV 1000 mg q8h + RBT 150 mg/d or 300 mg 2×/wk NFV 1000 mg tid + RBT 150 mg/d or 300 mg 2×/wk RTV—standard + RBT 150 mg qod EFV—standard + RBT 450–600 mg/d NVP 200 mg bid + RBT 300 mg 2×/wk RTV + SQV standard + RBT 150 mg 2–3×/wk or 300 mg/wk LPV/r-standard + RBT 150 mg qod SQV & DLV—no data • Contact with INH-resistant strain: Rifamycin + pyrazinamide × 2 mo as noted above

Table 15. (continued)

Disease	Indications: Start and Stop*	Preferred Regimen (cost/mo)	Comment/Alternative
P. carinii pneumonia	*Start prophylaxis:* Prior PCP CD4 <200/mm³ Thrush or FUO *Stop prophylaxis:* Primary* prophylaxis when CD4 >200/mm³ × 3 mo Secondary prophylaxis when CD4 >200 × 6 mo	TMP-SMX 1 DS/d ($4.20/mo) or 1 SS/d	• Alternatives: TMP-SMX 1 DS 3 d/wk; dapsone 100 mg/d; regimens for toxoplasmosis (see below), aerosolized pentamidine 300 mg/mo ($100/mo + administration costs) or atovaquone 750 mg bid with meals ($612/mo) • Safety of discontinuation of prophylaxis is well confirmed (NEJM 2001;344:159; NEJM 2001;344:168)
Toxoplasmosis	*Start prophylaxis:* CD4 <100/mm³ *plus* positive serology (IgG) *Stop prophylaxis:* Primary prophylaxis*—stop when CD4 >200/mm³ × 3 mo Secondary prophylaxis*—stop when CD4 >200 × ≥6 mo, asymptomatic & completed initial Rx	TMP-SMX 1 DS/d ($2.10/mo)	• Main issue is use of alternative regimens in patients with TMP-SMX intolerance: Dapsone 50 mg/d + pyrimethamine 50 mg/wk + leucovorin 25 mg/wk or dapsone 200 mg/wk + pyrimethamine 75 mg/wk + leucovorin 25 mg/wk or atovaquone 1500 mg/d ± pyrimethamine 25 mg qd + leucovorin 10 mg/d • Immune reconstitution: Data are inadequate to support discontinuation of secondary prophylaxis
M. avium complex	*Start prophylaxis:* CD4 <50/mm³ *Stop prophylaxis:* Primary prophylaxis*—stop	Clarithromycin 500 mg bid ($207/mo) Azithromycin 1200 mg 1 ×/wk ($126/mo)	• Alternatives are rifabutin 300 mg/d or rifabutin 300 mg/d + azithromycin 1200 mg q wk (see dose adjustments for rifabutin and for PI/NNRTIs under TB prophylaxis prior page)

	when CD4 >100/mm³ × 3 mo Secondary prophylaxis*—stop when CD4 >100 × ≥6 mo + 12 mo Rx + asymptomatic		• A disadvantage of clarithromycin is possible resistance to clarithromycin, which is the favored agent for treatment of established infection • Immune reconstitution: Data strongly support discontinuation of primary prophylaxis (NEJM 2000;342:1085; Ann Int Med 2000;133:493) and discontinuation of secondary prophylaxis (AIDS 1999;13:1647; AIDS 2000;14:383)
Varicella	Exposure to chickenpox or zoster and no history of chickenpox or shingles or negative VZV antibody	Varicella-zoster immune globulin (VZIG) 625 units (5 vials) IM ≤96 hr after exposure	• Acyclovir prophylaxis is no longer advocated because of no supporting data
GENERALLY RECOMMENDED			
Streptococcus pneumoniae	CD4 count >200	Pneumococcal vaccine 0.5 mL IM × 1 ($11)	• Response is reduced in patients with CD4 counts <200/mm³ • Revaccination sometimes advocated with vaccination >5 yr ago or vaccination when CD4 <200/mm³ + immune reconstitution
Influenza	All patients: Consider category	Influenza vaccine ($4.50)	• CDC guidelines are ambivalent. Favoring vaccination is one report showing influenza may have a worse course in HIV-infected patients and evidence that it works in this population. Against use is slight transient elevation in viral load and poor response in persons with CD4 counts <200/mm

Table 15. (continued)

Disease	Indications: Start and Stop*	Preferred Regimen (cost/mo)	Comment/Alternative
Hepatitis B	Negative anti-HBc screening test	HBV vaccine × three doses at 0, 1, and 6 mo ($161)	• Measure anti-HBsAg level at 1–6 mo after third dose; if <10 IU/mL repeat series
Hepatitis A	HCV infection + neg anti-HAV	HAV vaccine × 2 at 0 & 6 mo	None
PRIMARY PROPHYLAXIS NOT RECOMMENDED FOR MOST PATIENTS			
CMV	CD4 <50/mm³ + positive CMV serology	Oral ganciclovir 1000 mg tid ($1440/mo)	• Concerns for primary prophylaxis are cost, promotion of ganciclovir resistance, and variations in supporting data
CMV retinitis	*Stop prophylaxis:* Secondary prophylaxis*—stop when CD4 >100–150/mm³ + no evidence active disease + regular opthal exams		• Recurrences with high CD4 counts have been reported (JID 2001;183:1285) • Largest study showed recurrences in 2/48 and "immune recovery vitritis in 9 (AIDS 2001;15:23)
Candida	CD4 <100/mm³	Fluconazole 100–200 mg/d ($217–$434/mo)	• Efficacy established for prevention of cryptococcosis and *Candida* esophagitis (and thrush) • Concerns are cost, lack of evidence for prolongation of survival, and promotion of infection with azole-resistant *Candida* spp

Cryptococcosis	CD4 <50/mm³ *Stop prophylaxis*—stop when CD4 count >100–200/mm³ × ≥6 mo + completed initial Rx *Secondary prophylaxis*: completed initial Rx + asymptomatic	Fluconazole 100–200 mg/d ($217–$434/mo)	• Efficacy established • Concerns are failure to show survival advantage, promotion of azole-resistant *Candida* and *C. neoformans*, drug interactions, infrequency of cryptococcosis, and cost
Histoplasmosis	CD4 <100/mm³ plus endemic area *Stop prophylaxis*—no recommendations *Secondary prophylaxis*—no recommendations	Itraconazole capsules 200 mg/d or suspension 100 mg/d ($390/mo)	• Efficacy established • Itraconazole capsules at this dose does not effectively suppress *Candida* infections
Coccidioidomycosis	CD4 <50/mm³ plus endemic area *Stop prophylaxis*—no recommendations *Secondary prophylaxis*—no recommendations	Fluconazole 400 mg/d ($868/mo)	• Efficacy of prophylaxis is unknown
Bacteria	Neutropenia ANC <500/mL	G-CSF 5–10 µg/kg SC qd × 2–4 wk or GM-CSF 250 µg/m² IV × 2–4 wk ($8000/mo)	

APV, amprenavir; EFV, efavirenz; IDV, indinavir; LPV/r, lopinavir + ritonavir; NFV, nelfinavir; NVP, nevirapine; RTV, ritonavir; SQV, saquinavir; DLV, delavirdine.
* Primary prophylaxis means no prior disease with designated pathogen; secondary prophylaxis means prior disease with indicated pathogen.

Table 16. Recommendations for Primary and Secondary Opportunistic Infection Prophylaxis during Pregnancy

P. carinii	Standard guidelines should be followed Some may choose to delay prophylaxis until after the first trimester Should use full dose of TMP-SMX (1 DS/d) owing to increased blood volume TMP-SMX, dapsone, aerosolized pentamidine considered safe
S. pneumoniae	Pneumovax may be given safely in pregnancy
Toxoplasmosis	Delay primary prophylaxis with pyrimethamine (category C)*-containing regimens owing to risk associated with this drug and low probability of toxoplasmosis; with secondary prophylaxis, most would continue pyrimethamine because of high rate of relapse when drug is stopped TMP-SMX (category C)* prophylaxis is acceptable
M. avium	Azithromycin is preferred for MAC prophylaxis (Obstet Gynecol 1998;91:165). Clarithromycin is teratogenic in animals and must be used in pregnancy with caution Rifabutin has had limited experience in pregnancy For secondary prophylaxis use azithromycin and ethambutol
Herpes simplex	Acyclovir is controversial for use in pregnancy, but experience of the registry is that it is safe (MMWR 1993;42:806)
Tuberculosis	INH is preferred for prophylaxis. It should be given with pyridoxine. Some would delay initiating INH until after the first trimester Chest x-ray should be done with appropriate lead aprons Experience with rifampin is limited, but it appears safe Pyrazinamide should be avoided because of lack of information
Varicella-zoster	Zoster immune globulin is not contraindicated in pregnancy and should be given to a susceptible pregnant woman after exposure
Fungal infection	Fluconazole (category C)* has been associated with fetal deaths and fetal abnormalities in animal studies with doses >20 × those used in people (CID 1996;22:336). Itraconazole shows embryotoxicity and teratogenicity in pregnant animals. Amphotericin B is preferred when fungal therapy is needed
Hepatitis B vaccine	Safe in pregnancy
Influenza vaccine	Safe in pregnancy

* FDA categories: A, controlled studies show no risk; B, no evidence of risk in humans; C, risk cannot be excluded, but potential benefits may outweigh risk; D, positive evidence of risk; X contraindicated in pregnancy.

Table 17. Recommendations for Vaccines in HIV-Infected Patients[a]

Vaccine	Indication/Category	Regimen (Cost[b])	Comment
Routine vaccinations			
Pneumococcal vaccine	All patients	0.5 mL IM ($11.90)	Risk of *S. pneumoniae* infection is increased 100-fold Antigenic response is best when CD4 count is >200/mm³ Revaccination consideration: >5 yr since prior vaccination or vaccination when CD4 < 200/mm³ + immune reconstitution
Influenza vaccine	All HIV patients in Oct-Dec (BIII)	0.5 mL IM ($4.37)	Risk of influenza (acquisition or severity) is possibly increased. Prevention may avoid complicated diagnostic evaluation of flu-like complaints Vaccination may increase HIV viral burden, transiently, but significance is not considered important

Table 17. (continued)

Vaccine	Indication/Category	Regimen (Cost[b])	Comment
Hepatitis B vaccine	All susceptible (negative anti-HBc test) patients (BII)	3 IM doses at 0, 1, and 6 mo Recombivax 10 μg Engerix 20 μg ($55.78/dose or about $165 for the series)	Screening test is anti-HBc Risk of becoming HBsAg carrier is increased with HIV infection Measure antibody response at 1–6 mo after third-dose; nonresponders should receive repeat series
Hepatitis A	All susceptible (negative anti-HAV test) + chronic HCV	1-mL doses at 0 and 6 mo ($46/dose)	Risk of fulminant hepatitis with acute HAV in patients with chronic HCV infection About 30% of U.S. adult population has serologic evidence of prior HAV Many recommend HAV vaccination for all HIV-infected patients
Travel associated vaccines			
Oral polio	Contraindicated	—	Live vaccine; eIPV preferred If inadvertently given to household contact, contact should be avoided for 1 mo

Inactivated polio (eIPV)	Travel to developing countries for those without prior immunization	0.5 mL SC ($14.00)	Preferred polio vaccine for HIV-infected persons and close contacts. Polio has been eliminated from Western hemisphere
Yellow fever	Contraindicated		Live vaccine. With travel to endemic area advise patient of risk, instruct in control of mosquito exposure, and provide vaccination waiver letter
Japanese B encephalitis	Travel >1 mo to epidemic area	1 mL SC ×3 at days 0, 7, and 30 ($200)	Expensive and frequent side effects (not unique to HIV-infected persons)
Typhoid (ViCSP)	Travel to risk area (Latin America, Asia, Africa)	0.5 mL IM × 1 ($32.44)	Live attenuated Ty21a vaccine (Vivotif) is contraindicated. ViCSP is more expensive and no more effective than the parenteral inactivated vaccine but causes fewer side effects and requires only one dose
Typhoid inactivated vaccine	As above	0.5 mL SC × 2 separated by 1 mo ($10.16/20 doses)	

Table 17. (continued)

Vaccine	Indication/Category	Regimen (Cost[b])	Comment
Hepatitis A	Travel to developing countries Gay men, injection drug users, chronic HCV infection (see above)	1 mL adult formulation IM × 1 ≥14 days before travel ($60 single dose)	Havrix may be used in place of immune globulin Serologic tests show 30% of adults are protected by prior infection
Cholera vaccine	Not recommended		No longer recommended or required
Other Vaccines			
Haemophilus influenzae type B	Not recommended	0.5 mg IM × 1 ($20.46/dose)	Not recommended because most infections with *H. influenzae* in HIV-infected persons involve nontypable strains (JAMA 1992; 268:3350)
Tetanus-diphtheria (Td) vaccine	All adults—booster q 10 yr	0.5 mg IM q 10 yr ($2.40)	HIV infection is not a contraindication

Measles, mumps, rubella (MMR) vaccine	Contraindicated	—	Live virus vaccine; one report of a serious reaction (MMWR 1995;43:959)
Varicella-zoster vaccine	Contraindicated	—	Live virus vaccine; over 90% of adults have serologic evidence of varicella infection; if HIV-infected person is seronegative—avoid contact with chickenpox and zoster
Lyme	Use if indicated	30 µg vaccine dose IM at 0, 1, and 12 mo ($184 for 3 doses)	Antibody levels fall rapidly. Concern for immune mediated arthritis (Med Lett 1999;41:29)

[a] Recommendations of Advisory Committee on Immunization Practices (MMWR 1993;42(RR-4)) and USPHS/IDSA committee on prevention of opportunistic infections (MMWR 1999;48(RR-10)).
[b] Average wholesale price (Medi Span, Hospital Formulary Pricing Guide, February 1999).

6—Antiretroviral Therapy
Management of HIV-Infected Patients
and Post-Exposure Prophylaxis

Historical Perspective

Three nearly simultaneous developments revolutionized HIV care during 1995–97. First, it was shown that HIV replicated at a rate that produced 10 billion virions daily throughout most of the disease (Nature 1995;373:117, 223). Second quantitative plasma HIV RNA was introduced as a method to determine prognosis and response to therapy. The third development was the introduction of new and more potent antiretroviral agents, protease inhibitors, and non-nucleoside reverse transcriptase inhibitors. HAART was popularized in 1996, and by 1997 the following were down by 60–80%: Hospitalizations, deaths, AIDS-defining diagnoses, etc. However, enthusiasm was tempered with the same tough issues with the new therapy: 1) There was still no cure; 2) no studies clearly defined when treatment should start; 3) there was substantial evidence that HAART was associated with severe consequences, especially lipodystrophy and mitochondrial toxicity; 4) clinical experience showed convincingly that adherence was critical to achieve virologic success—in fact the threshold for virologic failure in >50% was consumption of <95% of prescribed pills; and 5) increasing concern about resistance to antivirals both in treated patients and in newly infected patients. The result is a revision in the philosophy of care (Fig. 2) that is 1) more conservative in the recommendations for initiation of treatment, 2) still aggressive in use of HAART, 3) increasingly emphasizing adherence and regimen simplification, and 4) paying substantial attention to side effects.

Current Recommendations

The following recommendations are from the Panel on Use of Antiretroviral Agents in Adults and Adolescents of the Department of Health and Human Services (DHHS) and Kaiser Family Foundation (KFF) (revised version February 5, 2001, www.hivatis.org) and the International AIDS Society—USA (JAMA 2000;283:381). Note that recommendations for antiretroviral agents change rapidly, and the most recent DHHS/KFF version is available from the HIV/AIDS Treatment Information Service website (www.hivatis.org). The tables presented here are from the July 2001 version with material from Bartlett JG. *2001–2002 Management of HIV Infection,* www.hopkins-aids.edu. Chapter 6 is organized as follows:

A. Management of HIV-infected patients

A. MANAGEMENT OF HIV-INFECTED PATIENTS
When to Start Antiretroviral Therapy

Table 18. Indications for Initiation of Antiretroviral Therapy
DHHS Recommendations

Clinical Category	CD4+ T Cell Count and HIV RNA	Recommendation
Acute HIV syndrome or ≤6 mo of seroconversion	Any value	Treat
Symptomatic (AIDS, severe symptoms)	Any value	Treat
Asymptomatic	CD4 >350/mm³ VL <20,000 copies/mL (bDNA) or <55,000 copies/mL (RT-PCR)	Many experts would defer; 3-yr risk of AIDS diagnosis defining is <15%
Asymptomatic	CD4 >350/mm³ VL >30,000 copies/mL (bDNA) or >55,000 copies/mL (RT-PCR)	Some experts would treat because risk of an AIDS-defining complication within 3 yr is >15% Some experts will not treat but would follow the CD4 count closely
Asymptomatic	CD4 200–350/mm³ VL—any value	Treatment usually offered. Benefit of therapy has been shown only for CD4 <200/mm³; 3-yr probability of AIDS-defining diagnosis with CD4 200–350/mm³ + VL <20,000 (RT-PCR) is <15%
Asymptomatic	CD4 <200 VL—any value	Treat

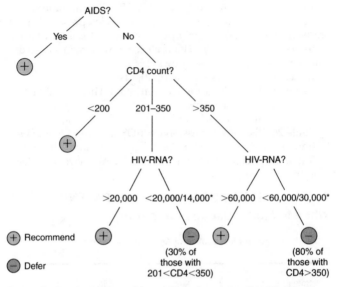

Figure 2. Treatment based on additional analysis of MACS data (Ann Intern Med 1997;126:946). Recommendation to initiate antiretrovirals in patients is defined by a 15% risk of an AIDS-deficiency diagnosis within 3 yr if untreated (courtesy of A. Munoz). *Male/female viral load levels based on data from NEJM 2001;344:720.

Table 19. Initial Treatment
IAS-USA Recommendations (JAMA 2000;283:381)

- Acute HIV syndrome
- Symptomatic chronic HIV infection
- Treatment based on CD4 count and viral load

	Viral Load		
	<5000 copies/mL	5000–30,000 copies/mL	>30,000 copies/mL
<350/mm³	Treat	Treat	Treat
350–500/mm³	Consider	Treat	Treat
>500/mm³	Defer	Consider	Treat

Table 20. Risk of Progression to AIDS-defining Illness (1987 Definition) Based on Baseline CD4 Cell Count and Viral Load[a]

CD4 ≤350 Plasma Viral Load (copies/mL)[b]		% AIDS (AIDS-defining Complication)[c]			
bDNA	RT-PCR	n	3 yr	6 yr	9 yr
501–3000	1501–7000	30	0	18.8	30.6
3001–10,000	7001–20,000	51	8.0	42.2	65.6
10,001–30,000	20,001–55,000	73	40.1	72.9	86.2
>30,000	>55,000	174	72.9	92.7	95.6
CD4 351–500 Plasma Viral Load					
501–3000	1501–7000	47	4.4	22.1	46.9
3001–10,000	7001–20,000	105	5.9	39.8	60.7
10,001–30,000	20,001–55,000	121	15.1	57.2	78.6
>30,000	>55,000	121	47.9	77.7	94.4
CD4 >500 Plasma Viral Load					
≤500	≤1500	110	1.0	5.0	10.7
501–3000	1501–7000	180	2.3	14.9	33.2
3001–10,000	7001–20,000	237	7.2	25.9	50.3
10,001–30,000	20,001–55,000	202	14.6	47.7	70.6
>30,000	>55,000	141	32.6	66.8	76.3

[a] Data from Multi-Center AIDS Cohort Study (MACS) (Ann Intern Med 1997;126:946).
[b] MACS numbers reflect plasma HIV RNA values obtained by bDNA testing. RT-PCR values are consistently 2- to 2.5-fold higher than bDNA values as indicated.
[c] AIDS was defined according to 1987 CDC definition and does not include asymptomatic individuals with CD4+ T cells <200/mm^3.

What to Start with

Table 21. Recommendations for Initial Antiretroviral Regimen from Three Sources

A. DEPARTMENT OF HEALTH AND HUMAN SERVICES
  • *Strongly Recommended* (one from column A and two from column B)*

A	B
Efavirenz	d4T + 3TC
Indinavir	d4T + ddI**
Nelfinavir	AZT + ddI
Ritonavir + saquinavir	AZT + 3TC
Ritonavir + indinavir	3TC + ddI
Liponavir + ritonavir	

  * Strongly recommended on basis of efficacy and quality of life issues.
    Efficacy evaluation is based primarily on: 1) controlled clinical trials
    comparing test regimen vs an alternative recommended regimen, 2) 24
    (preferably 48) wk data, 3) analysis based on virologic outcome for
    <400–500 copies/mL and <20–50 copies/mL, 3) analysis by intent-to-
    treat and as treated analysis, 4) separate analysis for baseline VL
    >100,000 copies/mL, 5) adequate sample size, and 6) toxicity data.
    Quality of life issues include toxicity, convenience of regimen, pill burden,
    etc.
  ** ddI + d4T should be avoided or given with caution during pregnancy
    owing to concern about lactic acidosis.

  • *Alternatives for column A:*
    Abacavir, amprenavir, nevirapine, delavirdine, ritonavir, nelfinavir +
    saquinavir-soft gel caps, saquinavir-soft gel caps
  • *Alternatives* for column B: AZT + ddC
  • *No recommendation:* Insufficient data for ritonavir + amprenavir, ritonavir
    + nelfinavir, hydroxyurea
  • *Should not be used:*
    Saquinavir-hard gel caps
    Column B: d4T + AZT, ddC + 3TC, ddC + d4T, ddC + ddI

B. INTERNATIONAL AIDS SOCIETY—U.S. (JAMA 2000;283:381)
  • *Recommendation*
    2 NRTIs* + PI or 2 PIs
    2 NRTIs* + NNRTI
    2 NRTIs* + 2 PIs
  • *Under evaluation*
    3 NRTIs (AZT + 3TC + ABC)
    NNRTI + PI + NRTI
  *AZT + ddI, AZT + 3TC, AZT + ddC, d4T + ddI, 3TC + d4T

C. *MEDICAL LETTER* CONSULTANTS
  (Med Lett 2000;42:1)
  • *Drugs of choice*
    2 NRTIs + 1 NNRTI (EFV often preferred)
    2 NRTIs + PI
    2 NRTIs + 2 PIs
  • *Alternatives*
    2 NRTIs + ABC
    2 PIs + NRTI + NNRTI
    2 PIs (full doses)
    PI + NNRTI + NRTI

Table 22. Relative Merits of Antiretroviral Treatment Regimens

Regimen	Advantage	Disadvantage
2 NRTIs + one PI	Standard Extensively studied regimens ± food requirements Durability >3 yr (Merck 035 trial) Genetic barrier to resistance NNRTI-sparing	Cross-resistance among PIs Inconvenience: bid or tid Toxicity: GI intolerance Lipid abnormalities Agent-specific ADRs
2 NRTIs + NNRTI	Comparable with standard (possibly better—EFV) Durability (≥2 yr) PI-sparing Pharmacologic barrier to resistance Good CNS penetration Convenience of qd dosing (EFV)	Cross-resistance among NNRTIs Toxicity CNS (EFV) Rash Lipid abnormalities (?) Hepatotoxicity (NVP)
ABC + 3TC + AZT	PI- and NNRTI-sparing Comparable with standard (but may show high failure rate with high baseline viral load) Simplicity of single pill bid	Limited experience May have suboptimal response with high baseline viral load Potential for extensive NRTI resistance Hypersensitivity reactions (ABC)
2 NRTIs + 2 PIs	Pharmacologic benefit with reduced doses and longer dosing intervals (regimen dependent) Increased potency (?) Improved tolerance Genetic and pharmacologic barrier to resistance	Cross-resistance among PIs Toxicity: GI intolerance, lipid abnormalities, agent-specific ADRs Complex drug interactions with multiple agents
2 NRTIs + PI + NNRTI	Increased potency (?) Reduced probability of resistance (?)	Risk resistance to all three classes Toxicity: ADRs of all three classes Complex drug interactions with multiple agents
NNRTI + 1 or 2 PIs	Avoid NRTI toxicity	Limited experience

Table 23. IAS-USA Guidelines (JAMA 2000;283:381)

Reason to Change	New Regimen
• Toxicity or intolerance	
VL achieved or <8–16 wk	Change implicated drug
VL not achieved and >8–16 wk	Change entire regimen or use resistance testing
• Virologic failure	
VL above target at 8–16 wk	Continue or intensify Confirm adherence
VL above target at 24–36 wk	Change entire regimen or use resistance testing
• Adherence problems	
VL achieved or <8–16 wk	Change to simplified regimen
VL not achieved at >8–16 wk	Change entire regimen or use resistance testing

When to Change Therapy

The goal of antiretroviral therapy is to reduce the level of HIV RNA to as low a level as possible for as long as possible, preferably using antiretroviral regimens that preserve future options, are relatively free of side effects, and are tailored to individual patient needs for adherence.

Analysis of virologic results from many studies indicates that the post-treatment viral burden nadir is the best predictor of the durability of a sustained viral response. Optimal results are achieved with undetectable virus using an assay with a threshold of 20–50 copies/mL. Studies show that <5% of all AIDS-defining complications occur in patients with a viral burden of <5000 copies/mL, suggesting that thresholds that define virologic failure and clinical failure may be different. However, the assumption is that virologic failure will spawn resistance, which may be problematic to the individual patient and lead eventually to clinical failure and to society in the evolution of resistance in wild-type virus (defined as the dominant strain in the infected population). Unfortunately, clinical studies show that only 15–30% of patients in most clinics achieve a level of <400–500 copies/mL for >1 yr. Based on these observations, most authorities consider a reduction to <20–50 copies/mL to be the ultimate goal of therapy, but this goal may be unrealistic in many patients. A concern is that the attempt to achieve unrealistic virologic responses may severely limit future therapeutic options because of the evolution of resistance to multiple agents.

The probability of achieving the goal of <50 copies/mL can be crudely predicted by the decay slope in plasma HIV RNA levels, which should show <500 copies/mL by 12 wk and <50 copies/mL at 16–24 wk. It should be emphasized that the ability to achieve these goals is highly contingent on the baseline viral load. Once the goal of therapy has been achieved, therapy should be continued indefinitely with monitoring of HIV RNA levels at 3- to 4-mo intervals and CD4 counts at 3- to 6-mo intervals.

A major goal of antiretroviral therapy is viral suppression as indicated by HIV RNA levels. Changes in therapy based on inadequate virologic response should be confirmed using at least two viral load measurements at a time of clinical stability, bearing in mind that the 95% confidence interval for the test is about 3-fold. The CD4 count usually follows the viral load changes with incremental increases based on the extent of HIV suppression (CID 2001;32:1231). Discordant changes occur in up to one-third of patients (JID 2001;183:1328). In most cases, therapeutic decisions are based on viral load responses rather than CD4 counts, although the CD4 count is probably a better indicator of susceptibility to an AIDS-deficiency complication.

Concepts in Antiretroviral Therapy

Blips.   Blips are transient elevations in viral load to detectable levels. They are seen in 40–50% of patients who achieve levels of <50 copies/mL. The implication is a borderline VL and a higher risk of subsequent virologic failure, but a change in therapy is not indicated.

Intensification.   Intensification is addition of a drug to intensify a virologic response that is good but not as profound as desired. This may be early in the viral decay cure (at 8–12 wk) or could occur with confirmed slight elevations after verologic success.

Structured Treatment Interruption.   There are five different types of interruption.

1. Discontinuation of unsuccessful therapy because of resistance accompanied by a high viral load. This is often associated with a rapid decline in CD4 count and return of PI susceptible HIV that may respond to therapy (NEJM 2001;344: 472).
2. Discontinuation of therapy in a patient who had a detectable virus for a sustained period. The goal is to allow reappearance of the virus to reimmunize the patient to HIV. Initial results with this tactic are good when initial treatment was during acute infection (Nature 2001;407:532); it has been generally less impressive when conducted in chronically infected patients.
3. Intermittent therapy or "structured intermittent treatment" in which there are scheduled treatment interruptions such as 1 wk on, then 1 wk off or 2 mo on and 1 mo off. The goal is to control the virus and reduce side effects and cost.
4. A variation in structured intermittent treatment is to suspend treatment when the CD4 count exceeds $350/mm^3$ and restart when it decays below that level. Thresholds in this approach are arbitrary.
5. Interrupted treatment for the first trimester of pregnancy for concern about the effects of these drugs on fetal organ formation.

Fitness.   The concept is that multiply mutated HIV strains may have reduced replicative capacity. The implication is that antiretroviral agents in the face of multiple resistance mutations and virologic failure may achieve clinical benefit despite the bad numbers. Evidence to support the concept is the rapid decline in CD4 count that accompanies return of wild-type HIV when failed therapy is stopped (NEJM 2001;344:472).

Multidrug Rescue.   Five to six drugs, arbitrarily selected and often recycled, are used in patients who have failed therapy. Supporting trials are sparce, and tolerance of these regimens is often poor.

Viral Load and CD4 Disconnect.   The failure of the expected inverse correlation of the viral load and CD4 count appears to apply to up to 35% of patients and is largely unexplained (Ann Intern Med 2000;133:401; JID 2000;181:946).

Virologic Failure.   All definitions are arbitrary. Most clinicians want a viral load of <50 copies/mL, most clinical cohort studies define viral failure at 400–500 copies/mL and most opportunistic infections viral load occur when viral load is >5000 copies/mL.

B. RECOMMENDATIONS FOR ANTIRETROVIRAL THERAPY IN PREGNANCY

Prevention of Perinatal Transmission—ACTG 076

ACTG 076 showed that AZT reduced the rate of perinatal transmission from 22.6% to 7.6% (NEJM 1996;335:1621). Multiple uncontrolled studies have confirmed the benefit of AZT in reducing perinatal transmission (JID 1995;172:353; CID 1995;20:1321), and subsequent surveillance studies in the U.S. showed substantial declines in the rates of perinatally acquired HIV that accompanied use of AZT in pregnant women (MMWR 1997;46:1986). Initial recommendations for women were based on ACTG 076 and were designed to prevent perinatal transmission only using the following three-part protocol (MMWR 1994;43(RR-11):1–20).

· **Before delivery.** AZT (300 mg bid, 200 mg tid, or 100 mg 5×/day) initiated at 14–34 wk of gestation and continued to onset of labor
· **During labor.** AZT (loading infusion of 2 mg/kg IV for 1 hr followed by continuous infusion 1 mg/kg/hr until delivery)
· **Infant.** AZT for the newborn (AZT syrup at 2 mg/kg every 6 hr) for the first 6 wk of life beginning 8–12 hr after birth

Antiretroviral Pregnancy Registry

Care providers with HIV-infected pregnant women treated with AZT, ddI, ddC, d4T, 3TC, ABC, nevirapine, efavirenz, ritonavir, amprenavir, saquinavir, or indinavir should report observations to the following:

Antiretroviral Pregnancy Registry
115 North Third Street, Suite 306
Wilmington NC 28401
Tel: 800-258-4263 or 910-251-9087
Fax: 800-800-1052

C. POST-EXPOSURE PROPHYLAXIS FOR HEALTH CARE WORKERS

Risk for Transmission

A total of 23 studies of needlesticks among health care workers demonstrate HIV transmission in 20 of 6135 (0.33%) exposed to an HIV-infected source (Ann Intern Med 1990;113:740). With mucosal surface exposure, there was one transmission in 1143 exposures (0.09%), and there were no transmissions in 2712 skin exposures. As of June 2000, there were 56 health care workers in the U.S. who had occupationally acquired HIV infection as indicated by seroconversion in the context of an exposure to an HIV-infected source. There are an additional 138 health care workers who had possible occupationally acquired HIV; these latter health care workers did not have documented seroconversion in the context of an exposure. Of the 56 confirmed cases, 1) the major occupations were nurses (23), laboratory technicians (19), and physicians (6); 2) all transmissions involved blood or bloody body fluid except for three involving laboratory workers exposed to HIV viral cultures; 3) exposures were percutaneous in 46, mucocutaneous in five, and both in two; and 4) to date there are no confirmed seroconversions in surgeons and no seroconversions with exposures to a suture needle.

PHS Recommendations for Post-exposure Prophylaxis (PEP)

Step 1. Determine exposure code (p 77)
Step 2. Determine HIV status code (p 78)
Step 3. PEP recommendations based on exposure category (EC) and HIV RNA level in the source (p 79)
Comments regarding recommendations follow.

- **Drug selection.** The only drug with established merit for reducing HIV transmission with needlestick injuries is AZT (Retrovir). The rationale for recommending AZT plus 3TC (lamivudine) is based on the greater antiretroviral activity of this combination when given to patients with established infection. The addition of a protease inhibitor reflects greater antiviral potency with the recommendation for high-risk injuries and settings in which resistance to

AZT and/or 3TC is anticipated based on the treatment regimen of the source. The preference for indinavir or nelfinavir is based on tolerance, bioavailability, and drugs available in 1997. The issue of drug selection has become more complex owing to the availability of 14 antiretroviral agents, concerns about toxicity, and concern about resistance in the source strain. Thus, in practice, these recommendations remain reasonable for many heath care workers with exposure from a source who has unknown serostatus, is untreated, or has a sensitive strain. If the source is known to have virologic failure while receiving antiretroviral drugs, the options are the standard regimen or a regimen based on established or suspected susceptibilities in the source with three exceptions: Efavirenz, nevirapine, and abacavir should usually be avoided because they cause serious reactions such as hepatoxicity (nevirapine), hypersensitivity (abacavir), or cognitive problems (efavirenz); in each case the reactions are most common in the first month of treatment (which represents the entire course of treatment).

- **Side effects.** Side effects according to the PEP Registry with 492 occupational exposures managed with standard CDC recommended regimens follow: nausea—57%, fatigue—38%, headache—18%, vomiting—16%, diarrhea—14%. The number who discontinued prophylaxis because of toxicity was 54% (Infect Control Hosp Epidemiol 2000;21:780). Stavudine (d4T) is an appropriate alternative for those who do not tolerate AZT, although AZT is the only drug with established efficacy. There are few side effects with 3TC. The major risks with indinavir are GI intolerance (10%) and renal calculi (0.8% with treatment for 1 mo). Recipients of indinavir must take >48 oz of fluid daily to reduce the probability of renal calculi.
- **Pregnancy testing.** Some facilities require a pregnancy test before administration of AZT post-exposure prophylaxis in female health care workers with childbearing potential.
- **Timing.** Prophylaxis should be initiated as rapidly as possible after exposure, preferably within 1–2 hr. Animal studies show no benefit when treatment is delayed 24–36 hr (JID 1993;168:1490; N Engl J Med 1995;332:444); nevertheless, the CDC recommends prophylaxis with a delay

of up to 1–2 wk with high-risk exposures. The Hopkins program includes a 72-hr "starter pack" to promote early prophylaxis when the health care worker is undecided. There is also a service to deliver initial doses to the operating room to prevent the need to break scrub.

- **Monitoring.** HIV serology is performed at baseline, 6 wk, 12 wk, and 6 mo. We are aware of three health care workers who seroconverted at >6 mo after occupational exposure. For patients who receive post-exposure prophylaxis, the drug toxicity monitoring should include a CBC and hepatic and renal function tests at baseline and 2 wk after treatment is initiated.

Management of occupational exposure (MMWR 2001;50: RR-1)

General

Immediate care: Wash wounds and skin with soap and water; flush mucous membranes with water

Determine risk: 1. Type of fluid-blood, visibly bloody fluid, other potentially infectious fluid or tissue and concentrated virus

2. Type of exposure

Evaluate source: 1) Test source for HBsAg, anti-HCV and anti-HIV (rapid testing for HIV preferred)

2) Unknown source—access risk for HIV, HCV, HBV

3) Do not test discarded needles, syringes etc.

Evaluate exposed HCW: HBV vaccination & vaccine response

Hepatitis C Exposure

- HCW-test anti HCV + ALT at baseline and at 4–6 months post exposure
- HCV RNA test at 4–6 wks (optional)
- Confirm anti-HCV test with confirmatory test
- Risk with HCV infected source = 1.8%
- No prophylaxis recommended

Hepatitis B Exposure

- Risk: Source HBeAg positive 37–62%
     Source HBeAg negative 23–37%

- Follow-up tests: anti HBs at 1–2 mo after vaccine if vaccinated

Vaccine status healthcare worker	Features of source	
	HBs Ag Positive	Source unknown
Unvaccinated	HBIG* + vaccine (3 doses)	HBV vaccine (3 doses)
Vaccinated Responder** Non-responder	No Rx HBIG × 1 + vaccine series or HBIG × 2***	No Rx Rx as source positive if high risk
Antibody status unknown	Test anti-HBs • >10 mIU/ml—No Rx • <10 mIU/ml—HBIG × 1 + vaccine booster	

* HBIG = Hepatitis B Immune Globulin. Dose is 0.06 ml/kg IM. Give ASAP and ≤7 days
** Responder defined by antibody level ≥10 mIU/ml
*** HBIG + vaccine series preferred for non-responders who did not complete the 3 dose series; HBIG × 2 doses preferred if 2 vaccine series and no response

HIV Exposure

- Risk with HIV infected source: 0.3%
  Risk increased with large volume, deep injury, high viral load in source, visible blood on needle, needle in artery or vein
- Estimated efficacy of AZT prophylaxis: 79%
- Percutaneous Injuries

Exposure	Status of source		Unknown
	Low risk	High risk*	
Not severe solid needle superficial	2 drug PEP**	3 drug PEP**	Usually none; consider 2 drug PEP***
Severe Large bore, visible blood on device, needle in pt artery or vein	3 drug PEP**	3 drug PEP**	Usually none; consider 2 drug PEP***

* Low risk: Asymptomatic HIV or VL <1,500 c/ml
High risk: Symptomatic HIV, AIDS, seroconversion, high viral load
** Concern for drug resistance—start prophylaxis and consult expert
*** Consider 2 drug PEP if source high risk or exposure is from unknown source where HIV likely

- Mucocutaneous exposure*

| Exposure | Status of Source | | Unknown |
	Low risk**	High risk**	
Small volumes	Consider 2 drug PEP	2 drug PEP	Usually no PEP; consider 2 drug PEP***
Large volume	2 drug PEP	3 drug PEP	Usually no PEP; consider 2 drug PEP***

* Non-intact skin = dermatitis, abrasion, wound.
Low risk
** Low risk—asymptomatic or VL <1,500 c/ml
High risk: symptomatic HIV, AIDS, acute seroconversion, high viral load
*** Consider if source has HIV risk factors or exposure from unknown source where HIV likely

- Recommended regimens
    2 drug PEP: AZT + 3TC or 3TC + d4T or d4T + ddI
    3 drug PEP: Above plus indinavir, nelfinavir, efavirenz, abacavir, ritonavir, Fortovase, amprenavir, delavirdine or liponavir/ritonavir
    Modify according to anticipated or measured resistance in source strain
    Drugs to avoid: Nevirapine and ddC
- Monitoring
    HIV serology repeated at 6 wks, 3 months and 6 months
- Counseling of healthcare worker
    Tx prophylaxis: Safe sex or no sex esp during first 6–12 wks
    Pregnancy: Pregnancy should no preclude PEP, but should avoid efavirenz and combination of d4T + ddI
    Toxicity: Frequency of side effects—74%, most commonly nausea, fatigue, headache, vomiting, diarrhea (see Infect Control Hosp Epidemiol 2000;21:780)

Table 24. Antiretroviral Therapy in Pregnancy

Issue	Recommendation	Comment
Drugs AZT	Use as much 076 protocol as possible	AZT and NVP are only drugs with established merit for preventing perinatal transmission All three components of 076 protocol contribute AZT confers benefit even when viral load is <1000/mL (JID 2001;183:539) Appears to reduce transmission even when maternal strain is resistant (JID 1998;177:557)
3TC	Recent studies show efficacy with AZT	AZT + 3TC reduced perinatal transmission rate to 1.8% (JAMA 2001;285:2083)
d4T	Do not use with AZT Avoid use with ddI	Pharmacologic antagonism Concern is three deaths in pregnant women receiving ddI + d4T due to lactic acidosis
Hydroxyurea	Do not use	Category D
EFV	Some avoid use during first trimester	Concern is teratogenic effect in primates; note that other antivirals have not been tested in primates
NVP	Consider single dose ± AZT in pregnant woman who presents in labor	Established efficacy with single dose of delivery + one infant dose. Concern—hepatoxicity, rash, and resistance (AIDS 2000;14:Flll)
Protease inhibitors	Issues in comment	Class appears safe (J AIDS 2000;25:306) Concerns are • IDV: Hyperbilirubinemia and renal calculi in neonate (theoretical concern only) • Monitor glucose intolerance • Pharmacokinetics: Preliminary data suggest concern for plasma levels

Table 24. (continued)

Issue	Recommendation	Comment
NRTIs	Issues in comment	Concern about mitochondrial toxicity based on a report of eight cases in exposed infants (Lancet 1999;354: 1080). Analysis of >20,000 AZT exposed infants showed no significant evidence of toxicity (NEJM 2000;343:805)
Variables		
Viral load	Viral load should be <1000 copies/mL at delivery regardless of initial CD4 count or viral load.	Risk of transmission is directly related to viral load. <1K: <1%; 1–10K: 17%; 10–50K: 21%; 50–100K: 31%; >100K: 41% (NEJM 1999;341:394)
Breastfeeding	Contraindicated in developed world	Risk of HIV transmission is 16% (JAMA 2000; 223:638). Issues in developing world are more complex (JAMA 2000; 283:1167; JID 2001;183:206)
Interventions		
First trimester	Consider delay in initiating or suspending treatment	Concern is effect on organ development. ART is a risk-benefit decision
C-section	Advocated at 38 wk if viral load is >1000 copies/mL	European Mode of Delivery Study randomly assigned HIV-infected women to cesarean vs vaginal delivery. Rate of perinatal transmission: 3/176 (1.8%) with cesarean vs 21/200 (10.5%) in controls. Concerns: Maternal risks modestly increased (J AIDS 2001;26:236). HAART or benefit with viral load <1000/mL not addressed

7—Antiretroviral Agents

Table 25. Antiretroviral Drugs Approved by FDA for HIV

Trade Name	Generic Name (abbreviation)	Firm	FDA Approval Date
Retrovir	zidovudine, AZT	GlaxoSmithKline	Mar 1987
Videx	didanosine, ddI	Bristol-Myers Squibb	Oct 1991
Hivid	zalcitabine, ddC	Hoffman-La Roche	Jun 1992
Zerit	stavudine, d4T	Bristol-Myers Squibb	Jun 1994
Epivir	lamivudine, 3TC	GlaxoSmithKline	Nov 1995
Invirase	saquinavir, SQV, hgc	Hoffman-La Roche	Dec 1995
Fortovase	saquinavir, SQV, sgc	Hoffman-La Roche	Nov 1997
Norvir	ritonavir, RTV	Abbott Laboratories	Mar 1996
Crixivan	indinavir, IDV	Merck	Mar 1996
Viramune	nevirapine, NVP	Boehringer Ingelheim	Jun 1996
Viracept	nelfinavir, NFV	Agouron Pharmaceuticals	Mar 1997
Rescriptor	delavirdine, DLV	Pharmacia & Upjohn	Apr 1997
Combivir	zidovudine and lamivudine	Glaxo Wellcome	Sep 1997
Sustiva	efavirenz, EFV	DuPont Pharmaceuticals	Sep 1998
Ziagen	abacavir, ABC	GlaxoSmithKline	Feb 1999
Agenerase	amprenavir, APV	GlaxoSmithKline	Apr 1999
Kaletra	lopinavir/ritonavir (LPV/r)	Abbott	Sep 2000

Table 26. Nucleoside Analogs

Generic name:	Zidovudine (AZT, ZDV)	Didanosine (ddl)	Zalcitabine (ddC)	Stavudine (d4T)	Lamivudine (3TC)	Abacavir (ABC)
Trade name:	Retrovir	Videx and Videx EC	Hivid	Zerit	Epivir	Ziagen
How supplied	100 mg caps (300 mg tabs) IV vials 10 mg/mL 300 mg + 3TC 150 mg as Combivir 300 mg + 3TC 150 mg + abacavir 300 mg as Trizivir	Buffered tabs: 25, 50, 100, 150, and 200 mg Videx EC: 125, 200, 250, and 400 mg caps avail. Powder packet: 100, 167, and 250 mg	0.375 and 0.75 mg tabs	15, 20, 30, and 40 mg caps	150 mg tabs 10 mg/mL oral soln 150 mg with AZT 300 mg as Combivir 300 mg + ABC 300 mg + AZT 300 mg as Trizivir	300 mg tabs 20 mg/mL oral soln 300 mg + 3TC 150 mg + 300 mg AZT as Trizivir
Dosing recommendations	200 mg tid or 300 mg bid Combivir 1 tab bid Trizivir 1 tab bid	>60 kg tabs: 200 mg bid or 400 mg qd <60 kg tabs: 125 mg bid or 250 mg qd Powder: >60 kg, 250 mg bid <60 kg, 167 mg bid	0.75 mg tid	>60 kg: 40 mg bid <60 kg: 30 mg bid	150 mg bid or with AZT as Combivir tab bid Trizivir: 1 tab bid	300 mg bid Trizivir 1 tab bid
Oral bioavailability	60%	30%–40%	85%	86%	86%	83%

Food effect	None	Levels ↓ 55% Buffered: Take >1 hr before or >2 hr after meal Videx EC: Take >1/2 hr before or >2 hr after meal	None	None	None	None Alcohol ↑ ABC levels 41%
Serum half-life	1.1 hr	1.6 hr	1.2 hr	1.0 hr	3–6 hr	1.5 hr
Intracellular T½	3 hr	25–40 hr	3 hr	3.5 hr	12 hr	3.3 hr
CNS penetration (% serum levels)	60%	20%	20%	30–40%	10%	Good
Elimination	Metabolized to AZT Glucuronide (GAZT) Renal excretion of GAZT	Renal excretion—50%	Renal excretion—70%	Renal excretion—50%	Renal excretion—unchanged	Metabolized Renal excretion of metabolites—82%
Major toxicity Class toxicity*	Bone marrow suppression; anemia and/or neutropenia Subjective: GI intolerance nausea, headache, insomnia, asthenia	Pancreatitis Peripheral neuropathy GI intolerance nausea, diarrhea Videx EC has fewer GI side effects	Peripheral neuropathy Stomatitis	Peripheral neuropathy Pancreatitis	Minimal toxicity	Hypersensitivity (2–5%), with fever, nausea, vomiting, malaise, morbilliform cough rash**
Clinical monitoring	CBC 9 1–3 mo	Peripheral neuropathy	Peripheral neuropathy	Peripheral neuropathy	—	—

* Class toxicity: Lactic acidosis with hepatic steatosis is a rare but potentially life-threatening toxicity with use of this class.
** Hypersensitivity reactions to abacavir may be serious. Most have fever, and symptoms may resemble flu and usually occur in first 4 wk: drug should be discontinued. It should not be restarted because more severe symptoms may occur within hours and may cause death.

Table 27. Non-Nucleoside Reverse Transcriptase Inhibitors

Generic name:	Nevirapine	Delavirdine	Efavirenz
Trade name:	Viramune	Rescriptor	Sustiva
Form	200 mg tabs; 50 mg/5 ml oral susp	100, 200 mg tabs	50, 100, 200 mg caps
Dosing recommendations	200 mg po qd × 14 days, then 200 mg po bid	400 mg po tid	600 mg po qd at hs
Oral bioavailability	>90%	85%	42%
Food effect	No effect Take without regard to meals	No effect Take without regard to meals	Increased 50% with high fat meal; avoid after high fat meal
Serum half-life	25–30 hr	5.8 hr	40–55 hr
Elimination	Metabolized by cytochrome P-450 (3A inducer); 80% excreted in urine (glucuronidated metabolites, <5% unchanged), 10% in feces	Metabolized by cytochrome P-450 (3A inhibitor); 51% excreted in urine (<5% unchanged), 44% in feces	Metabolized by cytochrome P-450 enzymes (3A mixed inhibitor/ inducer); 14–34% excreted in urine, 16–61% in feces

Drug interactions	Induces cytochrome P-450 enzymes Contraindicated drugs: None PI interactions (see p 86) Nevirapine reduces ketoconazole levels 63% (not recommended); decreases methadone levels significantly; titrate methadone dose Drugs that reduce nevirapine levels: Rifampin 37% (not recommended), rifabutin 16% (no data on dose)	Inhibits cytochrome P-450 enzymes Contraindicated drugs: Terfenadine, astemizole, ergot derivatives, triazolam, midazolam, cisapride, rifabutin, rifampin, H₂ blockers, proton pump inhibitors, simvastatin, lovastatin Delavirdine increases levels of clarithromycin, dapsone, quinidine, warfarin, sildenafil Antacids and didanosine: Separate administration by >1 hr PI interactions (see p 86)	Inhibits and induces cytochrome P-450 3A4 enzymes Contraindicated drugs: Astemizole, midazolam, triazolam, cisapride, ergot alkaloids, terfenadine Possibly important drug interactions: Rifampin, rifabutin, clarithromycin, phenobarbital, carbamazepine, ethinyl estradiol, phenytoin, warfarin PI interactions (see p 86) Methadone: May decrease levels of methadone—monitor
Major toxicity Class toxicity*	Hepatotoxicity in 12-20%; most common during 1st 4 wk; may have hepatic necrosis Rash (15-30%) may require hospitalization; rare cases of Stevens-Johnson syndrome	Rash; headaches	Dizziness, "disconnectedness," somnolence, insomnia, bad dreams, confusion, amnesia, agitation, hallucinations, poor concentration — 40%, usually resolves after 2 wk; take hs *Rash—severe in 5%; rare reports of Stevens-Johnson syndrome Teratogenic in cynomolgus monkeys. Some avoid in first trimester of pregnancy, and females should use adequate contraception methods
Clinical monitoring	Liver function tests q 1-2wk first 6 wk, then q 3 mo	—	—

* Class toxicity; Rash that may be severe; mechanism is not established; most common and severe with nevirapine.

Table 28. Protease Inhibitors

Generic name:	Indinavir	Ritonavir	Saquinavir		Nelfinavir	Amprenavir	Lopinavir/ ritonavir
Trade name:	Crixivan	Norvir	Invirase	Fortovase	Viracept	Agenerase	Kaletra
Form	200, 333, 400 mg caps	100 mg caps 600 mg/7.5 mL oral solution	200 mg caps	200 mg caps	250 mg tablets 50 mg/g oral powder	50, 150 mg caps 15 mg/mL oral soln	133 mg LPV + 33 mg RTV caps 80 mg LPV + 20 mg RTV/ mL oral soln
Usual dose	800 mg q 8h Separate buffered ddl dose by 1 hr	600 mg bid Separate buffered ddl dose by 2 hr	400 mg bid with ritonavir	1200 mg tid 1600 mg bid under study	750 mg tid or 1250 mg bid	1200 mg bid 1400 mg bid (oral soln)	400/100 mg (3 caps or 5 mL) bid
Food effect	Levels decrease 77%; take 1 hr before or 2 hr after meals; may take with low fat snack or skim milk	Levels increased 15%; take with food if possible to improve tolerability	No food effect when taken with RTV	Levels increase 6×; take with large meal unless taken with RTV	Levels increase 2–3×; take with meal or snack	High fat meal reduces AUC 20%; take with or without food but avoid high fat meal	Fat increases AUC 50–80%; take with food
Bioavailability	65% (on empty stomach)	Not determined	4%	Not determined	20–80%	Not determined, 14% lower with oral soln	Not known

Storage	Room temperature	Refrigerate caps Oral solution room temp	Room temperature	Room temperature or refrigerate	Room temperature	Room temperature	Room temp
Serum half-life	1.5–2 hr	3–5 hr	1–2 hr	1–2 hr	3.5–5 hr	7–10 hr	Lopinavir 5–6 hr
CNS penetration	Moderate	Poor	Poor	Poor	Moderate	Moderate	Not known
Elimination	Biliary metabolism cytochrome P-450 3A4 inhibitor	Biliary metabolism cytochrome P-450 3A4>2D6; 3A4 inhibitor	Biliary metabolism cytochrome P-450 3A4 inhibitor	Biliary metabolism cytochrome P-450 3A4 inhibitor	Biliary metabolism cytochrome P-450 3A4 inhibitor	Biliary metabolism cytochrome P-450 3A4 inhibitor	Biliary metabolism cytochrome P-450 3A4 inhibitor
Side effects	GI intolerance (10–15%); Nephrolithiasis or nephrotoxicity (10–20%); Headache; alopecia; dry skin and mucous membranes paronychia, hepatitis, thrombocytopenia, blurred vision Lab: Increase indirect bilirubinemia (inconsequential) Class side effect*	GI intolerance (20–40%); Paresthesias—circumoral and extremities (10%); taste perversion (10%); asthenia Lab: Increase triglycerides (60%), transaminase (10–15%), CPK, and uric acid Class side effects*	GI intolerance (10–20%); headache; transaminase increases Class side effects*	GI intolerance (20–30%); headache; transaminase increases Class side effects*	Diarrhea (10–30%) Class side effects** Increased transaminase	GI intolerance (10–30%) Rash (20–25% usually at 1–10 wk), Stevens-Johnson syndrome (1%) Paresthesias (10–30%—perioral or peripheral) Increased transaminase levels Class side effects*	GI intolerance esp diarrhea Asthenia Hepatitis Oral soln in 42% ETOH-disulfiram reaction

* Fat redistribution and lipid abnormalities have become increasingly recognized with the use of protease inhibitors. Fat redistribution is a cosmetic issue, and mechanism is unknown. Patients with hypertriglyceridemia or hypercholesterolemia should be evaluated for risks for cardiovascular events and pancreatitis. Possible interventions include dietary modification, lipid lowering agents, or discontinuation of protease inhibitors.

Table 29. Drugs That Should Not be Used with Protease Inhibitors or Non-Nucleoside Reverse Transcriptase Inhibitors*

Drug Category*	Indinavir	Ritonavir	Saquinavir	Nelfinavir	Delavirdine	Efavirenz	Amprenavir	Lopinavir
Cardiac	None	Amiodarone, encainide, flecainide, propafenone, quinidine	None	None	None	None	None	Flecainide, propafenone
Lipid lowering agents	Simvastatin, lovastatin	Simvastatin, lovastatin	Simvastatin, lovastatin	Simvastatin, lovastatin	Simvastatin, lovastatin	None	Simvastatin, lovastatin	Simvastatin, lovastatin
Anti-mycobacterial	Rifampin	Rifampin (?)	Rifampin, rifabutin	Rifampin	Rifampin, rifabutin	Rifampin	Rifampin	Rifampin
Ca++ channel blocker	None	Bepridil	None	None	None	None	Bepridil	None
Antihistamine	Astemizole, terfenadine	Astemizole, terfenadine	Astemizole, terfenadine	Astemizole, terfenadine	Astemizole, terfenadine	Astemizole, terfenadine	Astemizole, terfenadine	Astemizole, terfenadine

GI	Cisapride	Cisapride	Cisapride	Cisapride	Cisapride, H₂-blockers	Cisapride	Cisapride	Cisapride
Neuroleptic	None	Clozapine, pimozide	None	None	None	None	None	Pimozide
Psychotropic	Midazolam, triazolam	Midazolam, triazolam	Midazolam, triazolam	Midazolam, triazolam	Midazolam, triazolam	Midazolam, triazolam	Midazolam, triazolam	Midazolam, triazolam
Ergot alkaloid (vasoconstrictor)	Dihydroergotamine, ergotamine (various forms)	Dihydroergotamine, ergotamine (various forms)	Dihydroergotamine, ergotamine (various forms)	Dihydroergotamine, ergotamine (various forms)	Dihydroergotamine, ergotamine (various forms)	Dihydroergotamine, ergotamine (various forms)	Dihydroergotamine, ergotamine (various forms)	Dihydroergotamine, ergotamine (various forms)
Herbs	St. John's wort	St. John's wort	St. John's wort	St. John's wort	St. John's wort	St. John's wort	St. John's wort	St. John's wort

* Alternatives: Rifabutin (MAC)—clarithromycin, ethambutol, azithromycin; antihistamine—loratadine; psychotropic—temazepam, lorazepam; lipid-lowering—atorvastatin, pravastatin, fluvastatin.

Table 30. Drug Interactions That Require Dose Modifications or Cautious Use

Drugs Affected	Indinavir (IDV)	Ritonavir (RTV)	Saquinavir* (SQV)
ANTIFUNGALS Ketoconazole	Levels: IDV ↑ 68% Dose: IDV 600 mg tid	Levels: Keto ↑ 3× Dose: Use with caution Do not exceed 200 mg/d	Levels: SQV ↑ 3× Dose: Standard
ANTI-MYCO-BACTERIALS Rifampin	Levels: IDV ↓ 89% Contraindicated	Levels: RTV ↓ 35% Contraindicated	Levels: SQV ↓ 84% Contraindicated unless using RTV + SQV-rifampin 600 mg qd or 2–3 ×/wk
Rifabutin	Levels: IDV ↓ 32% Rifabutin ↑ 2× Dose: ↓ rifabutin to 150 mg qd IDV 1000 mg tid	Levels: Rifabutin ↑ 4× Dose ↓ rifabutin to 150 mg qd or dose 3×/wk; RTV standard dose	Levels: SQV ↓ 40% Not recommended
Clarithromycin	Levels: Clari ↑ 53% No dose adjustment	Levels: Clari ↑ 77% Dose adjust for renal insufficiency	Levels: Clari ↑ 45% SQV ↑ 177% No dose adjustment With RTV + SQV use clari 150 mg 2–3 ×/wk
ORAL CONTRACEPTIVES	Levels: Norethindrone ↑ 26% ethinylestradiol ↑ 24% No dose adjustment	Levels: Ethinyl estradiol ↓ 40% Use alternative or additional method	No data
ANTICONVULSANTS Phenobarbital Phenytoin Carbamazepine	Unknown but may decrease IDV levels substantially Use alt or RTV + IDV	Unknown Use with caution	Unknown but may decrease SQV levels substantially
METHADONE	No change in methadone levels	Methadone ↓ 37%, may require dose increase	No data

Table 30. (continued)

Drugs Affected	Nelfinavir (NFV)	Amprenavir (APV)	Lopinavir/ritonavir (LPV/r)
MISCELLANEOUS	Grapefruit juice ↓ IDV levels by 26% Sildenafil** Statins***	Desipramine ↑ 145%, reduce dose Theophylline ↓ 47%, monitor theo levels Many possible interactions (see product insert) Sildenafil** Statins***	Grapefruit juice increases SQV levels Dexamethasone decreases SQV levels Sildenafil** Statins***
ANTIFUNGALS Ketoconazole	No dose adjustment necessary NFV	Levels: Keto ↑ 44% APV ↑ 31%	Levels: Keto ↑ 3× LPV ↑ 13% Dose ?
ANTI-MYCO-BACTERIALS Rifampin	Levels ↓ 82% Contraindicated	Levels APV ↓ 82% Contraindicated	Levels: LPV ↓ 75% Avoid
Rifabutin	Levels: NFV ↓ 32% Rifabutin ↑ 2× Dose: ↓ rifabutin to 150 mg qd NFV ↑ to 1000 mg tid	Levels: APV ↓ 15% Rifab ↑ 193% Dose: ↓ rifabutin to 150 mg qd	Levels: LPV ↓ 17% RFB ↑ 3× Dose RFB 150 mg qod, LPV/r - standard
Clarithromycin	No data	Levels: APV ↑ 18% Clari NC Dose: Usual	No data
ORAL CONTRACEPTIVES	Levels: Norethindrone ↓ 18%, ethinylestradiol ↓ 47% Use alternative or additional method	Not studied Use alternative or additional method	Ethinylestradiol ↓ 42%; use alternative method
ANTICONVULSANTS Phenobarbital Phenytoin Carbamazepine	Unknown but may decrease NFV levels substantially; monitor levels	Unknown but may decrease amprenavir levels substantially; monitor levels	Unknown Use with caution
METHADONE	NFV decreases methadone levels substantially, but minimal effect on methadone maintenance dose—monitor	No data	Methadone ↓ 53% Titrate methadone dose
MISCELLANEOUS	Sildenafil** Statins***	Abacavir: APV ↑ 30% Sildenafil** Statins***	Sildenafil**

Table 30. (continued)

Drugs Affected	Delavirdine (DLV)	Efavirenz (EFV)	Nevirapine (NVP)
ANTIFUNGALS Ketoconazole	Not studied	Not studied	Keto ↓ 63% NVP ↑ 15–30% Not recommended
ANTI-MYCO- BACTERIALS Rifampin	Levels: DLV ↓ 96% Not recommended	Levels: EFV ↓ 25% No dose adjustment	NVP ↓ 37% Not recommended
Rifabutin	Levels: DLV ↓ 80% Rifabutin ↑ 100% Not recommended	EFV unchanged Rifabutin ↓ 35% Dose ↑ rifabutin to 450 mg/d or 600 mg 2–3 ×/wk EFV dose— standard	No data
Clarithromycin	Levels: Clari ↑ 100% DLV ↑ 44% Dose adjust for renal failure	Levels: Clari ↓ 39% Alternative recommended	Levels: Clari ↑ 26% Dose: Standard
ORAL CONTRACEPTIVES	No data Use alternative or additional method	Levels: Ethinyl estadiol ↑ 37% Use alternative method	Ethinyl estradiol ↓ 20%; use alternative method
ANTICONVULSANTS Phenobarbital Phenytoin Carbamazepine	Unknown but may decrease DLV levels substantially Monitor levels	Unknown Use with caution Monitor levels	Unknown Use with caution Monitor levels
METHADONE	No data	Methadone ↓ significantly Titrate methadone effect	Methadone ↓ significantly Titrate methadone effect
MISCELLANEOUS	May increase levels of dapsone, warfarin, and quinidine Sildenafil** Statins***	Monitor warfarin when used concomitantly	None

* Some drug interaction studies were conducted with Invirase. May not necessarily apply to use with Fortovase.
** Sildenafil (Viagra): Concurrent use with protease inhibitors or DLV increases sildenafil levels and may cause side effects. Do not exceed 25 mg/48 hr.
*** Statins: Potential for large increase in statin levels. Best options are atorvastatin and pravastatin.

Table 31. PI-PI Combinations and PI-NNRTI Combinations: Effect of Drugs on Levels (AUC)/Dose

Drug Affected	Ritonavir	Saquinavir	Nelfinavir	Amprenavir	Lopinavir	Nevirapine	Delavirdine	Efavirenz
Indinavir (IDV)	IDV 400 mg bid + RTV 400 mg bid or IDV 800 mg bid + RTV 100–200 mg bid	Insufficient data	Limited data for IDV 1200 mg bid + NFV 1250 mg bid	IDV 800 mg tid, APV 800 mg tid	IDV 600 mg bid LPV/r standard	IDV 1000 mg q8h, NVP standard	IDV 600 mg q8h DLV standard	IDV 1000 mg q8H EFV standard
Ritonavir (RTV)		Invirase or Fortovase 400 mg bid + RTV 400 mg bid or RTV 100 mg qd + SQV 1600 mg qd*	RTV 400 mg bid + NFV 500–750 mg bid	RTV 100–200 mg bid + APV 600 mg bid* or APV 1200 mg qd + RTV 200 mg qd	Co-formulated	Standard (both drugs)	No data	RTV 600 mg bid (500 mg bid for intolerance +) EFV 600 mg hs

Table 31. (continued)

Drug Affected	Ritonavir	Saquinavir	Nelfinavir	Amprenavir	Lopinavir	Nevirapine	Delavirdine	Efavirenz
Saquinavir (SQV)			NFV standard + Fortovase 800 mg tid or 1200 bid	SQV 800 mg tid, APV 800 mg tid* (limited data)	Fortovase 800 bid LPV/r standard	No data	Fortovase 800 mg tid, DLV standard (monitor transaminase levels)	Not recommended
Nelfinavir (NFV)				NFV 750 mg tid, APV 800 mg tid* (limited data)	No data	Standard (both drugs)	NFV 1250 mg bid + DLV 600 mg bid (limited data)	Standard (both drugs)
Nevirapine					LVP/r 533/133 mg bid NVP-standard (limited data)	No data	—	—
Efavirenz (EFV)				EFV standard + APV 1200 mg tid or APV 1200 mg bid + RTV 200 mg bid + EFV 600 mg qd	EFV standard LPV/r 533/133 mg bid	No data	No data	—

Adapted from DHHS guidelines (www.hivatis.com, June 2001).
* Added by author.

Table 32. HIV-Related Drugs with Overlapping Toxicities

Bone Marrow Suppression	Peripheral Neuropathy	Pancreatitis	Nephrotoxicity	Hepatotoxicity	Rash	Diarrhea	Ocular Effects
Chemotherapy	Didanosine	Cotrimoxazole	Adefovir	Delavirdine	Abacavir	Didanosine	Cidofovir
Cidofovir	Isoniazid	Didanosine	Aminoglycosides	Efavirenz	Amprenavir	Clindamycin	Ethambutol
Cotrimoxazole	Stavudine	Lamivudine	Amphotericin B	Fluconazole	Cotrimoxazole	Lopinavir	Rifabutin
Cytotoxic	Zalcitabine	(children)	Cidofovir	Isoniazid	Dapsone	Nelfinavir	
Dapsone		Pentamidine	Foscarnet	Itraconazole	NNRTIs	Ritonavir	
Flucytosine			Indinavir	Ketoconazole			
Ganciclovir			Pentamidine	NNRTIs			
Hydroxyurea				NRTIs			
Interferon				Protease			
Primaquine				inhibitors			
Pyrimethamine				Rifabutin			
Ribavirin				Rifampin			
Sulfadiazine							
Trimetrexate							
Zidovudine							

Table 33. Mitochondrial Toxicity (AIDS 2000;14:2723)

Agents: d4T > ddl > AZT > ABC > 3TC

Lactic acidosis: Symptoms are wasting, abdominal pain, fatigue, and exercise-induced dyspnea
Lab tests: Lactic acid levels—normal <1.5–2 mmol/ml; sl elevation 2–5 mmol/ml, severe 5–10 mmol, life-threatening >10 mmol/ml.
Other lab changes are increased LDH, CPK, AST/ALT, CT scan of abdomen showing steatosis
Treatment: Withdrawal of NRTls or switch to NRTI regimen unlikely to cause this. Time required for normalization of lactic acid is an average of 50 days

Other consequences of mitochondrial toxicity (suspected associations)

Agent	Complication
AZT	Cardiomyopathy, marrow suppression with anemia or neutropenia, myopathy
d4T	Peripheral neuropathy
ddC	Peripheral neuropathy
ddl	Peripheral neuropathy and pancreatitis
All NRTls	Fat atrophy—extremities, buttocks, buccal fat (face)

Table 34. National Cholesterol Educational Program (JAMA 2001;285:2486) **LDL goal based on risk**

Risk	LDL Goal (mg/dL)	Drug Therapy LDL (mg/dL)**
*Coronary heart disease or other form of atherosclerotic disease or diabetes or multiple risks**	<100	>130 100–130: Prescription optional
Multiple risks >2 of 1) smoking, 2) HBP >140/90 or HBP meds, 3) HDL <40, 4) bad genes in first degree relative male with CHD <55, female <65, 5) age >45 male, >55 female	>130	10-yr risk 10–20%* >130 10-yr risk <10%* >160
Risk factor 0–1	<160	>190 160–189: Prescription optional

* Determined by a complicated point system that factors age, cholesterol, HDL, and systolic BP.
** Major interventions are therapeutic life-style changes (TLC) and drugs. TLC emphasizes diet with reduced saturated fat (<7% total calories) and cholesterol (<200 mg/d). Other TLCs are exercise, weight reduction, increased fiber (16–25 g/d) and LDL lowering plant stanols/sterols (2 g/d).

Triglycerides (must be fasting level)
Normal level: <150 mg/dL
High level: 200–499 mg/dL
Very high levels: >500 mg/dL
Very high levels mandate immediate intervention to prevent pancreatitis and to reduce risk of cardiovascular disease. Two interventions:
1) Very low fat diet (<15% calories), weight reduction, and exercise and 2) drug therapy with fibrate or nicotinic acid

Table 35. Treatment of Hyperlipidemia—ACTG Guidelines (CID 2000;31:1216)

Lipid Problem	Preferred	Alternative	Comment
Isolated high LDL	Statin*	Fibrate**	Start low doses and fibrate up; with PIs, watch for myopathy
High cholesterol and triglycerides	Statin or fibrate	Start one and add other	Combination may increase risk of myopathy
High triglycerides	Fibrate**	Statin*	

* Statin: Pravastatin 20 mg/d (maximum dose 40 mg) or atorvastatin 10 mg/d (maximum dose 80 mg/d).
** Fibrate: Gemfibrozil 600 mg bid ≥30 min before meal or micronized fenofibrate 200 mg qd.

NUCLEOSIDE ANALOGUES

AZT (Zidovudine)

Trade name: Retrovir (GlaxoSmithKline)

Forms.   100 mg caps and 300 mg tabs; IV vials with 10 mg/mL (20 mL); 300 mg in combination with lamivudine (3TC) as Combivir; 300 mg in combination with lamivudine (3TC) and abacavir (ABC) as Trizivir

Cost. $1.86/100 mg tab; $5.57/300 mg; $10.33/Combivir tab; $16/Trizivir tab

Financial assistance.   800-722-9294

Dose regimens

Standard—200 mg PO tid or 300 mg bid or 1 Combivir bid or 1 Trizivir bid

Hepatic failure—200 mg bid

Renal failure—creatinine clearance ≤10 mL/min or dialysis 300 mg/d

Pregnancy—300 mg bid, 200 mg bid, or 100 mg 5 × /d; delivery—2 mg/kg/hr × 1 hr, then 1 mg/kg/hr until delivery; infant received 2 mg/kg PO q6h × 6 wk (MMWR 1994;43[RR-1]: 1)

Post-exposure in health care workers—200 mg po tid or 300 mg po bid × 4 wk (MMWR 1995;44:929)

HIV-associated dementia—200–400 mg po q2–5×/d (600–1200 mg/d)

Renal failure—Creatinine-clearance 10–50 mL/min: 300 mg bid; <10 mL/min: 100 mg q8–12h

Hepatic failure—standard dose

Pharmacology

Bioavailability—60%; $T_{1/2}$serum: 1.1 hr; $T_{1/2}$ serum with renal failure: 1.4 hr; $T_{1/2}$ intracellular: 3 hr; CNS penetration: 60%

Elimination—metabolized to AZT glucuronide that is renally excreted as G-AZT

Note: AZT has superior CNS penetration compared with alternative nucleoside analogues; this may be an important factor in selection of drugs used in patients with dementia

Monitoring.   CBC q3mo or more frequently with anemia or leukopenia

Note nearly all patients develop clinically inconsequential macrocytosis within 4 wk of initiating AZT. The lack of macrocytosis should raise concern about compliance.

Side effects

Subjective complaints—headache, malaise, GI intolerance, insomnia, and/or asthenia—dose related and may resolve with continued treatment. GI intolerance is especially common and may improve with AZT administration with food and/or more frequent dosing.

Marrow suppression—with anemia and/or neutropenia. Frequency and severity related to dose, duration, and stage. Management: Reduce dose or discontinue with Hgb ≤7.5 g/dL or absolute neutrophil count (ANC) <750–1000/mm^3; alternative is co-administration of G-CSF or EPO, respectively.

Miscellaneous—*myopathy* with increased CPK; *hepatitis* with increased transaminase levels; *cardiomyopathy* with reduced LV function by ECHO (association with AZT is unclear); *fingernail discoloration* (common and unimportant)

Lactic acidosis and hepatic steatotosis—class reaction

Drug interactions

Marrow suppression—concurrent use with ganciclovir and other marrow-suppressing agents is usually contraindicated. Use with caution and monitor CBC carefully with dapsone, TMP-SMX, flucytosine, interferon, sulfadiazine, hydroxyurea, and amphotericin.

Miscellaneous—there is antagonism in vitro and in vivo when used in combination with d4T (stavudine). Concurrent use is contraindicated. Methadone increases AZT levels 30–40%; there is no effect on methadone levels (J AIDS 1998;18:435).

Pregnancy.   Category C

The National Cancer Institute reported in January 1997 that administration of AZT in doses 12–15 × those used in patients proved carcinogenic to the offspring of pregnant mice. A second study by GlaxoSmithKline using doses equivalent to those used in patients showed no carcinogenic potential in pregnant mice. NIH subsequently convened a panel to review these data. The unanimous conclusion was that the established benefits of AZT for preventing perinatal transmission outweigh the hypothetical risk. A subsequent report from France suggested mitochondrial toxicity with neurologic sequelae in children exposed to AZT in utero (Lancet 1999;354:1084) This prompted a large scale evaluation of 20,000 infants exposed to AZT in utero that showed no evidence of immunologic, oncogenic, cardiac, or neurologic consequences (NEJM 2000;343:805).

ddI (Didanosine)

Trade name: Videx and Videx EC (Bristol-Myers-Squibb)

Forms.   *Buffered tabs:* 25, 50, 100, 150, and 200 mg. The 200 mg tabs are formulated for once daily dosing (400 mg qd). *Powder packets* of 100, 167, and 250 mg; *Videx EC* is an enteric coated capsule without buffer for once daily administration: 125, 200, 250, and 400 mg. Advantages of Videx EC: 1) once daily administration, 2) improved GI tolerance (less diarrhea), and 3) avoidance of buffer-related drug interactions.

Cost.   Buffered tabs: 100 mg—$1.98; 200 mg—3.95; powder pack 250 mg—$4.93; Videx EC 400 mg cap—$9.53

Financial assistance.   800-272-4878

Dose regimens

Standard—administration on an empty stomach

	Buffered Tabs[a]	Videx EC Caps	Powder
Food	>1 hr before or >2 hr after meal	>1/2 hr before or 2 hr after meal	≥1 hr before or ≥2 hr after meal
>60 kg dose	200 mg bid	400 mg qd	250 mg bid
<60 kg dose	125 mg bid	250 mg qd	167 mg bid

[a] Tabs must be chewed thoroughly or crushed and dissolved in water.

Renal failure—Creatinine clearance 10–50 mL/min: 50% standard dose; creatinine clearance <10 mL/min: 25% usual dose. A concern with renal failure is Na^+ (11.5 mEq/tab) and Mg^{++} (15.7 mEq/tab). With hemodialysis or peritoneal dialysis: 25%

Hepatic failure—consider dose reduction

Pharmacology
Bioavailability—30 to 40%

$T_{1/2}$ serum—1.6 hr; $T_{1/2}$ renal failure—3.1 hr; $T_{1/2}$ intracellular—25–40 hr; CNS penetration—20%

Elimination—renal: 50%

Monitoring.   Amylase q 1–2 mo is sometimes advocated, but utility of this practice for preventing severe pancreatitis is unclear; most important is to warn patient of symptoms of pancreatitis and peripheral neuropathy.

Side effects
Peripheral neuropathy—in 5–12% related to dose and duration. Management: discontinue ddI or reduce dose.

Pancreatitis—in 1–9%; risk with history of pancreatitis, advanced HIV, alcoholism, and concurrent medications that cause pancreatitis. Concurrent use with d4T and/or hydroxyurea may increase risk of pancreatitis. Management of pancreatitis—reduce dose or discontinue if routine monitoring shows amylase is ≥1.5–2 × upper limit of normal.

Gastrointestinal intolerance—Videx EC is better tolerated; methods to improve tolerance of buffered tabs are to dissolve tabs in ice water or apple juice or try powder form.

Miscellaneous—marrow suppression, hyperuricemia, hepatitis, rash, Na^+ load (11.5 mEq/tab and 60 mEq/powder packet); Mg^{++} load (15.7 mEq/tab)

Lactic acidosis and hepatic steatosis—class adverse effect

Drug interactions
Interactions from buffer in ddI formulations—drugs requiring gastric acidity should be given 2 hr before or 2 hr after ddI—indinavir, ritonavir, delavirdine, fluoroquinolones, dapsone, ketoconazole, itraconazole, and tetracyclines. (These interactions are not seen with Videx EC.)

Pancreatitis and neuropathy—drugs that cause pancreatitis should be used with caution: pentamidine, ethambutol, and alcohol. Drugs that cause peripheral neuropathy should be used with caution or avoided: cisplatin, ddC, d4T, disulfiram, ethionamide, INH, phenytoin, vincristine, hydralazine, metronidazole (long-term use only), and glutethimide.

Miscellaneous—methadone reduces AUC of ddI by 60%; ddI has no effect on methadone.

Pregnancy—category B; ddI and d4T should be avoided in pregnancy because of three deaths ascribed to lactic acidosis.

ddC (Dideoxycytidine)

Trade name: Zalcitabine (Hoffman-LaRoche)

Forms.   0.375 and 0.75 mg tabs

Cost. $2.60/0.75 mg tab

Financial assistance.   800-282-7780

Dose regimen

Standard—0.75 mg tid

Renal failure—creatinine clearance >50 mL/min—0.75 mg tid; 10–50 mL/min—0.75 mg bid; <10 mL/min—0.75 mg q 24h; dialysis—0.75 mg qd

Hepatic failure—standard dose

Pharmacology

Bioavailability—85%

$T_{1/2}$ serum—1.2–2 hr; $T_{1/2}$ intracellular—3 hr; CNS penetration—20%

Elimination—renal excretion 70%

Monitoring.   Warn patient of symptoms of peripheral neuropathy

Side effects

Peripheral neuropathy—17–31%, related to dose and duration. Management: Discontinue; patients with mild symptoms or symptoms that have resolved may be treated with half dose.

Miscellaneous—stomatitis, aphthous ulcers, pancreatitis, hepatitis

Drug interactions

Peripheral neuropathy—drugs that cause peripheral neuropathy should be avoided or used with caution—ddI, d4T, cisplatin, disulfiram, ethionamide, INH, phenytoin, vincristine, glutethimide, gold, hydralazine, and metronidazole

d4T (Stavudine)

Trade name: Zerit (Bristol-Myers-Squibb)

Forms.   15, 20, 30, and 40 mg caps; oral solution 1 mg/mL (200 mL) $3.86

Cost. $4.60/15 mg cap; $4.78/20 mg cap; $5.10/30 mg cap; $5.20/40 mg cap

Financial assistance.   800-272-4878

Dose regimen

Renal failure—Creatinine clearance

Wt.	>50 mL/min	10–50 mL/min	<10 mL/min
>60 kg	40 mg bid	20 mg q 12–24h	20 mg qd
<60 kg	30 mg bid	15 mg q 12–24h	15 mg qd

Dialysis—25% usual dose post-dialysis

Hepatic failure—standard

Peripheral neuropathy—dose reduction to 20 mg po bid or discontinue

Pharmacology

Bioavailability—86% (not influenced by food)

$T_{1/2}$ serum—1 hr; $T_{1/2}$ renal failure—8 hr; $T_{1/2}$ intracellular—3.5 hr; CNS penetration—30–40%

Elimination—renal 50%

Monitoring.   Warn patient of symptoms of peripheral neuropathy; warn of symptoms of pancreatitis if given concurrently with ddI

Side effects

Peripheral neuropathy—15–21%, related to dose and duration

Miscellaneous—pancreatitis, hepatitis, neutropenia

Class adverse effects—mitochondrial toxicity with lactic acidosis $\pm$ hepatic steatosis; fat atrophy

Drug interactions

D4T-AZT interaction—stavudine shows pharmacologic antagonism with AZT, presumably because of competition for intracellular phosphorylation. Concurrent use is contraindicated

Peripheral neuropathy—drugs that cause peripheral neuropathy should be avoided or used with caution: Ethionamide, ethambutol, INH, phenytoin, vincristine, glutethimide, gold, hydralazine, long-term metronidazole. Concurrent use with other nucleoside analogues that cause peripheral neuropathy (ddI and ddC) must be done with caution. Combination of d4T and ddI shows high incidence of peripheral neuropathy—up to 24% in some series (AIDS 2000;14:273). Reversible if drug is promptly discontinued

Methadone—concurrent use with methadone shows little effect on d4T levels and no effect on methadone levels

Monitoring. Warn patient about pancreatitis and peripheral neuropathy

Pregnancy. Category C; combination of ddI + d4T should be avoided in pregnancy because of three deaths ascribed to lactic acidosis

3TC (Lamivudine)

Trade name: Epivir (GlaxoSmithKline)

Forms. Oral solution with 10 mg/mL; 150 mg tabs lamivudine (3TC); 150 mg + AZT 300 mg as Combivir; 150 mg combined with AZT 300 mg and ABC 300 mg as Trizivir; 100 mg tabs for treatment of hepatitis B

Cost. $4.77/150 mg tab; $10.33/Combivir tab and $16/Trizivir tab

Financial assistance. 800-722-9294

Dose regimen
Standard for HIV—150 mg po bid
Standard for hepatitis B—100 mg/d × 52 wk

Renal Failure, CrCl Levels	HBV (mg/d)*	HIV (mg)**
>50 mL/min	100	150 bid
10–50 mL/min	100	150 qd
<10 mL/min	10–15	50 qd
Dialysis	10	25–50 qd

* Loading dose of 100 mg with CrCl >15 mL/min; <15 mL/min use 35 mg loading dose.
** Loading dose of 150 mg.

Hepatic failure—HIV: 50 mg qd

Hepatitis B virus is inhibited by lamivudine (NEJM 1995;333:1657); treatment of patients who were co-infected with HIV and HBV showed significant reduction in HBV DNA concentrations

(Ann Intern Med 1996;125:705). A 1-yr trial with 100 mg/d vs placebo showed that patients with chronic HBV infection had reduced rates of progression to fibrosis, enhanced elimination of HBV DNA, and clearance of HBVe Ag (NEJM 1998;339:61). Resistance by HBV is an anticipated problem (Lancet 1997;349:20).

Pharmacology. Oral bioavailability—86%; $T_{1/2}$ serum—3–6 hr; $T_{1/2}$ intracellular—12 hr; CNS penetration—10%; elimination—renal 71%.

Side effects. Minor: Headache, nausea, diarrhea, abdominal pain, and insomnia

Drug interactions.   None

Drug interactions.   TMP-SMX (1 DS/d) increases 3TC levels; significance is unknown

Pregnancy.   Category C

Abacavir (ABC)

Trade name: Ziagen (GlaxoSmithKline)

Form.   300 mg tabs; oral suspension with 20 mg/mL; 300 mg + 3TC 150 mg + AZT 300 mg as Trizivir

Cost. $6.41/300 mg tab; $16/Trizivir tab

Financial assistance.   800-722-9294

Dose regimens.
Standard—300 mg PO bid
Renal failure—no data but <20% excreted in urine; use standard dose
Liver failure—standard dose

Pharmacology
Bioavailability—83%, food—no effect, $T_{1/2}$—1.5 hr; intracellular $T_{1/2}$—3.3 hr; CNS levels are 27–33% of serum levels

Elimination—81% metabolized by alcohol dehydrogenase and glucuronyl transferase; metabolites are excreted in urine; 16% is recovered in stool, and 1% is unchanged in urine (metabolism does not involve cytochrome P-450 enzymes)

Side effects
Hypersensitivity reaction—a serious side effect reported in 2–3% of ABC recipients. Clinical features are fever (usually

>39°C), fatigue, malaise, GI symptoms (nausea, vomiting, diarrhea, abdominal pain), cough, and skin rash (maculopopular or urticarial) and may be difficult to distinguish from flu. Lab tests may show elevated liver function tests and CPK and lymphopenia. Rechallenge may be lethal. Most reactions occur within 6 wk of initiating treatment; median time of onset in one series was 9 days (Lancet 2000;356:1423). These reactions should be reported to the Abacavir Hypersensitivity Registry at 800-270-0425. Patients taking ABC should be warned of this reaction and should stop taking ABC if they develop typical findings. Rechallenge may be lethal; ≥3 lethal cases reported.

Miscellaneous—nausea, vomiting, malaise, headache, diarrhea, or anorexia

Lactic acidosis and steatosis—class reaction

Monitoring.   Warn patient regarding hypersensitivity reaction as a systemic reaction with fever, GI symptoms, and rash seen primarily in the first 6 wk of treatment. Warn not to rechallenge.

Drug interactions.   Alcohol increase ABC AUC 41% (AAC 2000;283:1811)

Pregnancy.   Category C

PROTEASE INHIBITORS

Saquinavir.   Trade name: Fortovase and Invirase (Hoffman-LaRoche)

Forms.   200 mg caps (soft gel capsules as Fortovase and hard gel capsules as saquinavir mesglate or Invirase)

Cost.   200 mg caps at $2.40 (Invirase); 200 mg caps at $1.23 (Fortovase)

Financial assistance.   800-282-7780

Dose regimen

Standard—Fortovase 1200 mg (six 200 mg caps) tid taken within 2 hr of a meal. Invirase is inferior owing to poor absorption and should be used only when combined with ritonavir. Usual regimen is Invirase or Fortovase (400 mg bid) plus ritonavir (400 mg bid). SQV is usually combined with RTV, which has the advantages of better pharmacokinetics, far more data substantiating efficacy, and avoidance of necessity to take with large meals.

Renal failure—standard

Hepatic failure—consider empiric dose reduction

Pharmacology

Bioavailability—4% for Invirase when taken with high fat meal to promote absorption; Fortovase is better absorbed (three-fold increase in AUC) and is given in double dose; food increases bioavailability. $T_{1/2}$ serum—1–2 hr; CNS penetration—poor

Elimination—96% biliary excretion via cytochrome P-450, 1% in urine

Side effects.   Dose-related GI intolerance with nausea, abdominal pain, and diarrhea in 20–30% (Fortovase) or 5–10% (Invirase); headache; hepatitis; hypolgycemia with type 2 diabetes (Ann Intern Med 1999;181:980)

Class adverse effects—lipodystrophy, insulin resistant hyperglycemia, osteoporosis

Monitoring—fasting lipid profile (cholesterol, LDH, HDL, triglycerides) and fasting blood glucose at baseline and at 3–6 mo; frequency of subsequent measurements depends on test results and other risk factors

Drug interactions

Drugs that are contraindicated for concurrent use—astemizole, cisapride, simvastatin, lovastatin, rifabutin, rifampin, ergot alkaloids, midazolam, terfenadine, and triazolam

Drugs affected by saquinavir—sildenafil ≤25 mg/48 hr

Drugs that reduce saquinavir levels—nevirapine, phenobarbital, phenytoin, dexamethasone, carbamazepine, and garlic

Drugs that increase levels of saquinavir—drugs that inhibit cytochrome P450 increase levels of saquinavir, including ketoconazole, itraconazole, fluconazole, ritonavir, indinavir, nelfinavir, and delavirdine

Rifampin/rifabutin—rifampin reduces SQV levels by 80%, and rifabutin reduces SQV levels 40%; these drugs should not be used concurrently. For TB use a non–rifamycin-containing regimen or change to an alternative PI

Combination with PI or NNRTIs

Ritonavir—RTV 400 mg bid + SQV (Invirase or Fortovase) 400 mg bid

Nelfinavir—NFV standard + Fortovase formulation (FTV) 800 mg tid

Delavirdine—DLV 600 mg tid + FTV 800 mg tid

Indinavir—combination not recommended

Efavirenz—combination not recommended

Nevirapine—combination not recommended

Amprenavir—APV 800 mg tid + FTV 800 mg tid (limited data)

Lopinavir/ritonavir—LPV/r 400/100 mg bid + FTV 800 mg bid

Indinavir. Trade name: Crixivan (Merck)

Forms.   200, 333 and 400 mg capsules

Cost. $2.78/400 mg cap

Financial assistance.   800-850-3430

Dose regimen

Standard—800 mg q8h in fasting state or with a light, non-fat meal. Patient should take >48 oz fluid/d to reduce frequency of nephrolithiasis. Store in original container with desiccant. A regimen that is commonly used to increase IDV levels and to avoid the inconvience of q8h dosing is 1) IDV 400 mg bid + RTV 400 mg bid or 2) IDV 800 mg bid + RTV 100–200 mg bid. The 400/400 mg regimen may be difficult for patients to tolerate; the 800/100–200 mg regimen may cause a higher rate of nephrolithiasis.

Renal failure—standard

Hepatic failure—600 mg q8h

Pharmacology

Bioavailability—absorption is best with fasting state or with a light meal that does not contain fat

$T_{1/2}$ serum—1.5–2 hr

Excretion—metabolized, especially hepatic glucuronidation and P-450-dependent pathways. Urine shows 5–12% unchanged drug and metabolites.

Side effects

Nephrolithiasis—hematuria in 10–28% depending on duration of treatment, age, and fluid prophylaxis (J Urol 2000;164: 1895). Renal stones are composed of indinavir precipitates. Incidence correlates with peak serum levels of indinavir; hydration and urinary pH are other factors. Should take 48 oz fluid daily, preferably at time of IDV administration. Indinavir may also cause interstitial nephropathy with proteinuria and renal failure.

Elevated indirect bilirubin—inconsequential increase in indirect bilirubin to >2.5 mg/dL without other changes in liver function tests in 10–15%

Miscellaneous—hepatitis with increased transaminase levels, headache, nausea, vomiting, diarrhea, metallic taste, fatigue, insomnia, blurred vision, dizziness, rash, thrombocytopenia, paronychia, ingrown toenails, dry skin, dry mouth, dry eyes

Class adverse effect—lipodystrophy, insulin resistant hyperglycemia osteoporosis (?)

Monitoring—serum creatinine and urinanalysis at 3- to 6-mo intervals. Fasting lipid profile (cholesterol, HDL, LDL, triglyceride) and blood glucose at baseline and at 3–6 mo; frequency of subsequent tests depends on initial results and concurrent risks

Drug interactions

Combinations with PIs and NNRTIs—RTV 100–200 mg bid + IDV 800 mg bid or RTV 400 mg bid + IDV 400 mg bid

Nelfinavir—NFV 1250 mg bid + IDV 1200 mg bid (limited data)

Amprenavir—APV 800 mg tid + IDV 1000 mg q8h

Efavirenz—EFV 600 mg qd + IDV 1000 mg q8h

Delavirdine—DLV 400 mg tid + IDV 600 mg q8h

Nevirapine—NVP 750 mg tid or 1250 mg bid + IDV 1000 mg q8h

Saquinavir—possible antagonism

Lopinavir/ritonavir—LPV/RTV 400/100 mg bid + IDV 600 mg bid

Rifampin/rifabutin—rifampin and rifabutin decrease levels of indinavir, and indinavir increases levels of rifabutin. Concurrent use with rifampin is contraindicated; rifabutin should be reduced to half dose (150 mg/d or 300 mg 2–3×/wk), and IDV is increased to 1000 mg tid.

Drugs that are contraindicated for co-administration—astemizole, cisapride, rifampin, simvastatin, lovastatin, St John's wort, midazolam, terfenadine, ergotamines, triazolam

ddI—buffered ddI given concurrently decreases indinavir absorption; these drugs should be given ≥2 hr apart or use Videx EC

Miscellaneous—ketoconazole and itraconazole increase IDV levels 70%; decrease IDV dose to 600 mg q8h. Clarithromycin levels increase 53%—no dose change. Ethinyl estradiol levels increase—no dose change. Anticonvulsants (phenobarbital, phenytoin, carbamazepine) may decrease IDV levels. Sildenafil (Viagra) levels increase 4 ×; maximum sildenafil dose is 25 mg/ 48 hr. Grapefruit juice decreases IDV 26%. Methadone interaction has not been studied.

Pregnancy. Category C

Ritonavir. Trade name: Norvir (Abbott)

Form. 100 mg caps; 600 mg/7.5 mL po

Cost. $2.06/100 mg cap

Patient assistance program. 800-659-9050

Dose regimen

Standard—600 mg bid PO; dose-escalation regimen days 1–2: 300 mg bid; days 3–5: 400 mg bid; days 6–13: 500 mg bid; day ≥14: 600 mg bid. With saquinavir, the ritonavir dose is 400 mg bid. Multiple other PIs are now used in combination with RTV (see drug interactions). Oral solution 600 mg bid = 7.5 mL bid; 400 mg bid = 5 mL bid.

Renal failure—standard

Hepatic failure—consider empiric dose reduction

Pharmacology

Bioavailability—60–80%

$T_{1/2}$ serum—3–5 hr

Excretion—hepatic metabolism by cytochrome P450 mechanism. Ritonavir induces its own excretion so that therapeutic levels are achieved with the graduated-dose regimen.

Side effects

GI intolerance—the major limiting side effect and sufficiently severe to require discontinuation of RTV in full doses in 10–30% (J AIDS 2000;23:236); often improves with treatment over 1 mo and with the graduated-dose regimen noted above; GI intolerance is dose related

Hepatotoxicity—RTV appears to cause drug induced hepatitis more frequently than other PIs (JAMA 2000;238:74). The lower doses used with PI combinations appear to cause less hepatotoxicity. Circumoral and peripheral paresthesias.

Lipodystrophy—fat redistribution, insulin resistant hyperglycemia, osteoporosis (?). RTV appears to cause more hypercholesterolemia than other PIs (J AIDS 2000;23:261; JAMA 2000;23:236)

Monitoring. Fasting lipid profile (cholesterol, LDL, HDL, triglycerides) and fasting blood glucose at baseline and 3–4 mo; frequency of subsequent tests depends on initial test results and concurrent risks.

Drug interactions

Drugs that are contraindicated for current use—astemizole, amiodarone, bepridil (Vascor), cisapride (Propulsid), clozapine, clorazepate (Tranxene), diazepam (Valium), encainide, ergot alkaloids, estazolam (Prosom), flecainide, flurazepam, lovastatin, meperidine (Demerol), midazolam (Versed), piroxicam (Feldene), pimozide, propoxyphene (Darvon), propafenone, quinidine, rifampin, simvastatin, terfenadine (Seldane), St John's wort, triazolam (Halcion), and zolpidem (Ambien)

Other interactions include increased levels of clarithromycin (CID 1996;23:6) (no dose change); induction of hepatic glucuronyl transferase and CYP1A2 activity results in reduced levels of theophylline and ethinyl estradiol—alternative methods of birth control should be used. Methadone levels are decreased 36%; consider dose increase. Desipramine levels are increased 145%; decrease desipramine dose. Buffered ddI reduces absorption of RTV, and the two drugs should be taken ≥2 hr apart or use Videx EC. Rifabutin levels are increased 4×, and the rifabutin dose should be reduced to 150 mg qod.

RTV—standard dose

Concurrent use with other PIs—ritonavir is usually combined with other protease inhibitors or non-nucleoside RT inhibitors to exploit the effect of RTV on levels of the second antiretroviral agent using the following regimens:

Saquinavir—RTV 400 mg bid + SQV 400 mg bid

Indinavir—IDV 800 mg bid + RTV 100–200 mg bid or IDV 400 mg bid + RTV 400 mg bid

Nelfinavir—NFV 500–750 mg bid + RTV 400 mg bid

Amprenavir—APV 600 mg bid + RTV 100 mg bid or APV 1200 mg qd + RTV 200 mg qd

Efavirenz—EFV 600 mg/d + RTV 500–600 mg bid

Nevirapine—standard doses

Delavirdine—no data

Pregnancy.   Category B

Nelfinavir. Trade name: Viracept (Agouron Pharmaceuticals)

Form.   250 mg tabs; 50 mg/g oral powder

Dose.   750 mg po tid or 1250 mg bid

Cost. $2.33/250 mg tab

Renal failure.   Standard

Hepatic failure.   Consider empiric dose reduction

Pharmacology

Bioavailability—20–80%; food increases absorption 2–3× $T_{1/2}$ serum: 3.5–5 hr

Excretion—hepatic cytochrome P-450, only 1–2% found in urine and up to 90% is found in stool primarily as oxidative metabolites

Side effects

In therapeutic trials, only 28 of 696 (4%) discontinued nelfinavir owing to side effects, usually because of diarrhea; 10–30% experience loose stools, and most respond to imodium.

Class adverse reaction—lipodystrophy; insulin resistant hyperglycemia; osteoporosis (?)

Monitoring.   Fasting lipid profile (cholesterol, LDL, HDL, triglycerides) and fasting blood glucose at baseline and at 3–6 mo; frequency of subsequent tests depends on results of baseline tests and associated risk factors.

Drug interactions

Drugs that must be avoided for concurrent use—cisapride, astemizole, midazolam, terfenadine, rifampin, St. John's wort, ergot alkaloids, and triazolam

Rifampin/rifabutin—rifampin reduces nelfinavir levels substantially and should not be given concurrently; rifabutin is not problematic for nelfinavir, but rifabutin levels increase 3-fold so that the rifabutin dose should be reduced to half (150 mg/d or 300 mg 2–3×/wk).

Interactions with other PIs—interactions are less pronounced compared with other agents in this class:

Indinavir—IDV 1200 mg bid + NFV 1250 mg bid

Ritonavir—RTV 400 mg bid + NFV 500–750 mg bid

Saquinavir—SQV (Fortovase) 800 mg tid or 1200 mg bid + NFV 1250 mg bid or 750 mg tid

Amprenavir—APV 800 mg tid + NFV 750 mg tid

Nevirapine—standard doses both drugs

Efavirenz—standard doses both drugs

Lopinavir/ritonavir—no data

Delavirdine—DLV 600 mg bid + NFV 1250 mg bid

Pregnancy.   Class B

Amprenavir (APV). Trade name: Agenerase (GlaxoSmith Kline)

Form.   50 mg caps; 150 mg soft gel caps; 15 mg/mL oral soln

Cost. $1.39/150 mg cap

Financial assistance.   800-722-9294

Dose standard.   1200 mg bid (eight 150 mg caps) given with or without food, but avoid high fat meal; oral soln 1400 mg bid

Renal failure—standard dose

Hepatic failure—moderate disease 450 mg bid; severe cirrhosis 300 mg bid

Pharmacology

Bioavailability—89%, AUC decreased 21% by concurrent high fat meal

$T_{1/2}$—7–9.5 hr

Elimination—hepatic metabolism CYP 3A inhibition is <RTV and comparable with IDV and NFV

Side effects

GI intolerance—nausea (15%), diarrhea (14%), vomiting (5%)

Miscellaneous—rash 11%, headache 6%, oral paresthesias 28%. APV contains large amounts of vitamin E (1744 units/d with 2400 mg daily dose); this with vitamin E supplement could produce bleeding diathesis.

Class adverse reactions—lipodystrophy, insulin resistant diabetes, osteoporosis?

Monitoring. Fasting blood lipids (cholesterol, LDL, HDL, triglycerides) and blood glucose at baseline and at 3–6 mo; subsequent tests at intervals based on these results and risks for diabetes or atherosclerosis.

Drug interactions

Drugs contraindicated for concurrent use—astemazole, bepridil, cisapride, ergotamines, lovastatin, midazolam, rifampin, terfenadine, St. John's wort, simvastatin, triazolam

Drugs that must be given with caution—amiodarone, carbamazepine, clozapine, lidocaine, phenobarbital, phenytoin, quinidine, tricyclics, warfarin, oral contraceptives (use alt methods)

Combination with other PIs and NNRTIs—

Indinavir—IDV 800 mg tid + APV 800 mg tid

Nelfinavir—NFV 750 mg tid + APV 800 mg tid

Fortovase—FTV 800 mg tid + APV 800 mg tid (limited data)

Efavirenz—EFV 600 mg qd + APV 1200 mg tid or APV 1200 mg bid + RTV 200 mg bid + EFV 600 mg hs

Ritonavir—RTV 100–200 mg bid + APV 600 mg bid or RTV 200 mg qd + APV 1200 mg qd or APV 1200 mg bid + RTV 200 mg bid + EFV 600 mg hs

Lopinavir/ritonavir—LPV/r 400/100 mg bid + APV 750 mg bid

Rifampin/rifabutin—rifampin reduces APV AUC 82% and should not be used concurrently. Rifabutin decreases APV AUC 15%, and APV increases RFB AUC 20%; use RFB 150 mg/d or 300 mg 2–3×/wk + APV standard dose.

Miscellaneous—clarithromycin increases APV AUC 32%; use standard dose of both drugs. Ketoconazole increases APV AUC 44%; dose implications are unclear.

Pregnancy. Category C

Lopinavir/ritonavir (LPV/r). Trade name: Kaletra (Abbott)

Form. Capsules with 133 mg lopinavir + 33 mg ritonavir; oral soln with 80 mg LPV + 20 mg RTV/mL

Cost. $3.76/133/33 mg cap

Financial assistance.   800-659-9050
Product information.   800-633-9110

Dose
Standard—400/100 mg bid (3 caps bid) with food
Renal failure—standard dose
Hepatic failure—consider empiric dose reduction

Pharmacology
Bioavailability: 80% with food; 48% with fasting; RTV is used only as a pharmacologic booster and not as an antiretroviral agent.

$T_{1/2}$ 5–6 hr

Elimination—metabolized by P450 CYP 3A4 isoenzymes. Less than 3% excreted in urine

Side effects
Gastrointestinal—most common, especially diarrhea that can usually be managed with immodium

Miscellaneous—hepatotoxicity in 10–12%; asthenia; oral solution has 42% ETOH giving possible disulfiram reaction

Class adverse reactions—lipodystrophy, insulin resistant hyperglycemia, osteoporosis?

Monitoring.   Fasting blood lipids (cholesterol, LDL, HDL, triglycerides) and blood glucose at baseline and at 3–6 mo; subsequent tests at intervals based on results and risks for diabetes or atherosclerosis

Drug interactions
Drug contraindicated for concurrent use—astemizole, cisapride, ergot derivatives, midazolam, lovastatin, pimozide, simvastatin, St John's wort

Drugs that require dose change—rifabutin 150 mg qod + LPV/r standard dose

Drugs to use with caution—ketoconazole levels increased 3×-? dose change; methadone AUC decreased 53%—monitor for withdrawal; ethinyl estradiol AUC decreased 42%—use alternate method; atorvastatin levels increase 6×—use with caution or use pravastatin or fluvastatin; anticonvulsants may decrease LPV levels—monitor anticonvulsant level; may increase sildenafil levels—do not exceed 25 mg/48 hr.

Dose adjustments with PIs and NNRTIs

Amprenavir—APV 750 mg bid + LPV/r 400/100 mg bid

Efavirenz—EFV 600 mg hs + LPV/r 533/133 mg bid

Indinavir—IDV 600 mg bid + LPV/r 400/100 mg bid

Nevirapine—NVP standard + LPV/r 533/133 mg bid

Saquinavir—Fortovase 800 mg bid + LPV/r 400/100 mg bid

Nelfinavir—no data

Delavirdine—no data

Pregnancy.   Category C

NON-NUCLEOSIDE REVERSE TRANSCRIPTASE INHIBITOR

Nevirapine. Trade name: Viramune (Roxane Labs)

Form.   200 mg tabs; 50 mg/5mL oral solution

Cost. $5.04/200 mg tab

Dose

Standard—200 mg qd ("lead in" ×2 wk), then 200 mg po bid unless rash precludes standard dose. If therapy is interrupted >7 days, then 200 mg dose should be restarted. May be given with or without food. Monitor liver function tests, especially during first 8 wk.

Renal failure—standard

Hepatic failure—consider empiric dose reduction

Pharmacology

Bioavailability—>90%; average is 93%; food has no effect, CSF penetration—45% of serum levels.

$T_{1/2}$—25 hr

Excretion—biotransformed by hepatic cytochrome P-450 enzymes. Nevirapine induces P-450, reducing its own half-life so that the half-life of 45 hr with early therapy is reduced to 25 hr.

Side effects

Hepatotoxicity—elevated transaminase levels to >5× ULN in 15–20%; may progress to hepatic necrosis requiring hepatic transplant or may be lethal. Most common in females and in first 8 wk. Patient should promptly report fever, rash, arthralgias, or GI symptoms, but most are asymptomatic.

Rash—seen in about 17%; usual rash is maculopapular and

erythematous with or without pruritus located on the trunk, face, and extremities. Most rashes are seen during the first month; 25% of patients in preclinical trials with rashes required hospitalization; and 7% of all patients required discontinuation of the drug. Indications to discontinue therapy are severe rash or rash accompanied by fever, blisters, mucous membrane involvement, conjunctivitis, edema, arthralgias, or malaise. Stevens-Johnson syndrome and three drug-associated deaths have been reported (Lancet 1998;351:567).

Miscellaneous side effects include fever, nausea, and headache.

Monitoring.   Monitor liver function tests—especially during first 8 wk; frequency is arbitrary. Warn of rash reaction. Need to monitor blood lipids and blood glucose is not established but is advised in patients at risk for atherosclerosis and diabetes.

Drug interactions.   NVP, like rifampin, induces P450 CYP3A4 isoenzymes resulting in enhanced metabolism of drugs metabolized by this mechanism. Clinically significant drug interactions are less frequent with NVP than with PIs and other NNRTIs. For example; few drugs are considered contraindicated for concurrent use, and most known drug interactions require only modest changes.

Not recommended for concurrent use—rifampin, ketoconazole

Drugs that show interactions—rifabutin decreases NVP levels 16%: no dose change; clarithromycin levels decrease 30% and NVP levels increase 26%: no dose change; ethinyl estradiol levels decrease 20%: use alternative method. Methadone levels decrease 60%: titrate methadone dose.

Pregnancy.   Class C

Delavirdine (DLV). Trade name: Rescriptor (Agouron)

Form.   100 and 200 mg tabs

Cost. $1.62/200 mg tab

Dose standard.   400 mg po tid. Food—minimal effect; ddI and antacids—take 1 hr apart

Renal failure—standard dose

Hepatic failure—consider dose reduction with severe liver disease

Pharmacology
Bioavailability—85%; CSF penetration poor (CSF; plasma = 0.02)

$T_{1/2}$—5.8 hr

Elimination—metabolized by cytochrome P-450 CYP 3A enzymes; delavirdine inhibits CYP 3A to increase its own levels and levels of IDV, NFV, SQV; 51% excreted in urine and 44% in feces

Side effects
Rash—18%; 4% require discontinuation; rash is diffuse, muculopapular, and red and on upper body. Stevens-Johnson syndrome reported and usually lasts 2 wk and resolves despite continuation of DLV. Discontinue if rash and fever, mucous membrane involvement, accompanying symptoms of swelling or arthralgias

Miscellaneous—headache

Monitoring.   Warn regarding rash reaction

Drug interactions
Drugs contraindicated for concurrent use—terfenadine, rifampin, rifabutin, ergot derivatives, astemizole, cisapride, midazolam, triazolam, H_2 blockers, proton pump inhibitors, simvastatin, lovastatin

Drugs with interactions requiring dose changes—clarithromycin levels increased 100%, and DLV levels increased 44%; adjust dose with renal failure; DLV may increase levels of dapsone, wafarin, and quinidine; for sildenafil do not exceed 25 mg/48 hr; take antacids and buffered ddI >1 hr apart or use Videx EC

Drugs that decrease levels of delavirdine—carbamazepine, phenobarbital, phenytoin, rifabutin, and rifampin

Concurrent use with PIs
Indinavir—IDV 600 mg q8h + DLV standard
Ritonavir—no data
Saquinavir—Fortovase 800 mg tid + DLV standard
Nelfinavir—NFV 1250 mg bid + DLV 600 mg bid
Amprenavir—no data
Lopinavir—no data

Pregnancy.   Category C

Efavirenz (EFV). Trade name: Sustiva (DuPont)

Form.   50, 100, 200 mg caps

Cost. $4.39/200 mg cap

Dose standard.   600 mg po hs

Renal failure—standard dose

Hepatic failure—consider empiric dose reduction

Pharmacology

Bioavailability—40–45% with or without food; high fat meals increase absorption 50% and should be avoided

$T_{1/2}$—40–55 hr; CSF 0.25–1.2% of serum levels

Elimination—metabolized by P-450 CY 3A4 isoenzymes; 14–34% excreted in urine as glucuronide metabolites and 16–61% excreted in stool

Side effects

CNS—noted in 52%, usually resolve in 2–3 wk and require discontinuation in 2–5%. Symptoms include confusion, abnormal dreams, dizziness, impaired concentration, and "depersonalization." Less common are hallucinations, somnolence, insomnia, amnesia, and euphoria. Patients should be warned, EFV is given at bedtime to reduce symptoms that are noted with the first day of therapy and may be confounded with alcohol or other psychoactive drugs.

Rash—about 15–27% develop rash that is usually morbilliform and usually does not require discontinuation. Rashes that are blistering or show desquamation are noted in 1–2%; Stevens-Johnson syndrome is reported in one of 2200 treated patients.

Hepatotoxicity—transaminase levels increase to $>5 \times$ ULN in 2–3%.

Lipid abnormalities—increase in cholesterol including increase in HDC; information about fat redistribution or diabetes is limited.

Teratogenicity—teratogenic in primates, so pregnant women should strictly avoid EFV, and women of childbearing potential should be warned. Note other antiretroviral agents have not been tested in primates, so it is unknown if this effect applies equally to other drugs.

Monitoring

CNS—patients must be warned of CNS effects that are anticipated with most patients, are usually apparent after the first dose, and usually resolve after 3 wk. Dose administration at bedtime is only partially effective in restricting symptoms to sleep time owing to long half-life of the drug. Particular caution is advised in patients with a history of mental illness, drug addition, or alcoholism and those receiving psychoactive drugs

Women of childbearing potential—warn of teratogenic effect of EFV and the need for adequate contraception, preferably with two forms. Some authorities recommend avoidance of EFV in women who are contemplating pregnancy, and some avoid the drug during the first trimester.

Lipodystrophy—EFV is commonly associated with an increase in cholesterol, including an increase in HDL. Effects on triglyceride levels, glucose levels, and fat redistribution are unknown; some authorities recommend monitoring analogous to that for PI recipients, i.e., fasting blood lipids and blood glucose at baseline and at 3–6 mo; subsequent tests depend on results of initial tests, risk factors, and results of ongoing trials.

Drug interactions

Drugs contraindicated for concurrent use—astemizole, midazolam, triazolam, cisapride, and ergot alkaloids

Drugs that decrease EFV levels—phenobarbital, phenytoin, and carbamazepine

Rifampin/rifabutin—EFV reduces rifabutin levels 35%; no effect of RFB on EFV levels. Use EFV 600 mg/d + RFB 450 mg qd or 600 mg 2–3×/wk, EFV standard dose. Rifampin decreases EFV levels 25%—no dose adjustment

Other interactions—when clarithromycin levels decrease 39% and the rate of rash reaction is increased—use alternative. When levels of ethinyl estradiol are increased 37%, use alternative. When methadone levels decrease, monitor for withdrawal; interaction with coumadin suspected; monitor anticoagulation

Interactions with PIs

Ritonavir—RTV 500–600 mg bid + EFV 600 mg/d

Nelfinavir—NFV 750 mg tid or 1250 mg bid + EFV 600 mg/d

Indinavir—IDV 1000 mg q8h + EFV 600 mg/d

Saquinavir—not recommended

Saquinavir + ritonavir—standard doses both drugs

Amprenavir—APV 1200 mg tid + EFV 600 mg hs or APV 1200 mg bid + RTV 200 mg bid + EFV 600 mg hs

Liponavir/ritonavir—LPV/r 533/133 mg (4 caps) bid + EFV 600 mg hs

Pregnancy. Category C

Some authorities recommend avoidance of EFV during first trimester.

MISCELLANEOUS AGENTS

Hydroxyurea (HU). Trade name: Hydrea (Bristol-Myers-Squibb)

Form.   500 mg caps

Cost. $1.30/500 mg cap

Dose standard.   500 mg bid

Note—HU is synergistic with ddI in vitro vs HIV. Only use when combined with ddI. HU also potentiates ddI toxicity with increased rates of pancreatitis and peripheral neuropathy

Pharmacology

Bioavailability—well absorbed

$T_{1/2}$—2–3 hr

Elimination—half is degraded by liver excreted as respiratory CO_2 and in urine as urea

Side effects

Marrow suppression—dose dependent suppression with anemia, leukopenia, and thrombocytopenia. Leukopenia is usually the first to occur and is the most common. Recovery is usually rapid when the drug is discontinued

GI intolerance—common and may be severe with nausea, vomiting, anorexia, diarrhea, and/or stomatitis

Pancreatitis—increase in rate of pancreatitis ascribed to ddI or ddI + d4T (AIDS 2000;14:273)

Dermatologic—rash, facial erythema, hyperpigmentation, oral ulceration, desquamation of face and hands, partial alopecia (J Am Acad Dermatol 1997;36:178)

Chronic leg ulcers—with treatment >3 yr (Ann Intern Med 1998;29:128)

Miscellaneous and rare—dysuria, neurologic complications (drowsiness, disorientation, hallucinations, convulsions), hyperuricemia, renal failure, fever, and chills

Monitoring.   Warn patient regarding risk and symptoms of peripheral neuropathy and pancreatitis; CBC at baseline and at 3- to 4-mo intervals. HU is contraindicated in pregnancy. Women of childbearing potential should be warned of teratogenic effects and should take two forms of contraception.

Drug interactions.   None

Pregnancy.   Category D

8—Management of Complications

Table 36. Management of HIV-Associated Complications

Opportunistic Infections (from Bartlett JG. 2001–2002 Medical Management of HIV Infection. Baltimore: Johns Hopkins University, Division of Infectious Diseases, 2001) (see www.hopkins-aids.edu)

	Preferred Regimen(s)	Alternative Regimen(s)	Comments
		FUNGAL INFECTION	
Pneumocystis carinii Acute Infection	Trimethoprim 15 mg/kg/d + sulfamethoxazole 75 mg/kg/d po or IV × 21 days (typical oral dosage is 2 DS tid)	Trimethoprim 15 mg/kg/d po + dapsone* 100 mg/d po × 21 days Pentamidine 4 mg/kg/d IV × 21 days (usually reserved for severe cases) Clindamycin 600 mg IV q8h or 300–450 mg po q6h + primaquine* 30 mg base/d po × 21 days Atovaquone 750 mg suspension po with meal bid × 21 days Trimetrexate 45 mg/m² IV day plus folinic acid 20 mg/m² po or IV q6h	In a comparative trial (ACTG 108) TMP-SMX, trimethoprim-dapsone, and clindamycin-primaquine were equally effective in patients with mild-moderate PCP (Ann Intern Med 124: 792, 1996) Intolerance to TMP-SMX is noted in 25–50%, primarily skin rash ± fever (Lancet 338:431, 1991)

117

Table 36. (continued)

	Preferred Regimen(s)	Alternative Regimen(s)	Comments
		FUNGAL INFECTION	
PCP (prophylaxis: U.S. Public Health/ IDSA guidelines (MMWR 48(RR-10), 1999; CID 30:S1, 2000) Initiation and discontinuation	TMP-SMX po 1 DS/day, 1 SS/ day	TMP-SMX1 DS 3×/wk Dapsone* 100 mg po qd Aerosolized pentamidine 300 mg q mo via Respirgard II nebulizer ± β₂ agonist (albuterol, 2 whiffs) Dapsone* 50 mg/d po plus pyrimethamine 50 mg/wk po plus folinic acid 25 mg/wk po or dapsone 200 mg plus pyrimethamine 75 mg plus leucovorin 25 mg po q wk Atovaquone 750 mg bid with meals Dapsone* 200 mg/wk po plus pyrimethamine 75 mg/wk po + folinic acid 25 mg/wk po	Patients with moderately severe or severe disease (PO₂ <70 mmHg or A-a gradient >35 mmHg) should receive corticosteroids (prednisone 40 mg po bid × 5 days, then 40 mg qd × 5 days, then 20 mg/d to completion of treatment). Side effects include CNS toxicity, thrush, *H. simplex* infection, tuberculosis, and other OIs (J AIDS 8:345, 1995) **Indications:** History of PCP, CD4 count <200–250/mm³ (or <14%), thrush, or unexplained fever >2 wk **Discontinuation:** Primary prophylaxis may be discontinued in patients with HAART when the CD4 count is >200/ mm³ × 3 mo (NEJM 339:1889, 1998; Lancet 353:201, 1999; Lancet 353: 1293, 1999). Patients with prior PCP (secondary prophylaxis) should also discontinue prophylaxis with these criteria (NEJM 344:159, 2001; NEJM 344:168, 2001)

Other regimens without established efficacy: Dapsone 50 mg/d po, pentamidine 4 mg/kg IM or IV q4wk, or Fansidar 1–2×/wk

TMP-SMX is superior in efficacy for PCP prophylaxis compared with dapsone and aerosolized pentamidine; TMP-SMX also prevents toxoplasmosis and bacterial infections (NEJM 332:693, 1995; NEJM 327:1842, 1992)

Adverse drug reactions requiring drug discontinuation are noted in 20–40% receiving TMP-SMX, 20–40% receiving dapsone, and 2–5% given aerosolized pentamidine

Patients who have mild or moderate reactions to TMP-SMX may be rechallenged or desensitized

Regimens that provide prophylaxis for PCP and toxoplasmosis are TMP-SMX, dapsone + pyrimethamine, and atovaquone (Ann Intern Med 122:755, 1997)

A CPCRA/ACTG trial showed atovaquone (750 mg bid) was as effective as dapsone (NEJM 339:1889, 1998)

Aspergillosis
Invasive pulmonary infection (CID 30: 696, 2000)

Amphotericin B 1.0–1.4 mg/kg/d ± 5-FC 100 mg/kg/d

Itraconazole 200 mg po bid with food (capsules) or 100–200 mg bid with empty stomach (liquid)

Itraconazole 200 mg IV bid × 4, then 200 mg IV qd

Amphotec 3–4 mg/kg/d IV

Abelcet 5 mg/kg/d IV

AmBisome 3–5 mg/kg/d IV

Caspofungin 70 mg IV × 1, then 50 mg IV/d

Total dose of amphotericin B: 30–40 mg/kg. Long-term maintenance is usually not necessary

Predisposing factors: Corticosteroids: decrease or stop if possible; neutropenia: G-CSF and avoid 5-FC

Recommendations based on IDSA guidelines (CID 30:696, 2000)

New preparations of amphotericin B include Abelcet, Amphotec, and AmBisome. Advantage is reduced nephrotoxicity and less infusion related reactions. Cost is >$400/treatment

Table 36. (continued)

	Preferred Regimen(s)	Alternative Regimen(s)	Comments
		FUNGAL INFECTIONS	
			Study by NIAID Mycosis Study Group showed response rate to itraconazole (200–400 mg/d) was 60% (Arch Intern Med 157:1857, 1997)
Candida Oropharyngeal (thrush) Initial infection (see HIV Clin Trials 1:47, 2000; CID 32:662, 2000)	Clotrimazole oral troches 10 mg 5×/day	Fluconazole 100 mg po qd Nystatin 500,000 units gargled 5×/day Amphotericin B oral suspension 1–5 mL qid swish and swallow Amphotericin B 0.3–0.5 mg/kg/d IV Itraconazole‡ 100 mg/d oral suspension	Treat until symptoms resolve (usually 10–14 days) Fluconazole is superior to ketoconazole with better efficacy, fewer drug interactions, more predictable absorption, but higher price. Itraconazole—use liquid formulation; efficacy comparable with fluconazole but more drug interactions (Am J Med 104:33, 1998) Amphotericin B (po or IV) and itraconazole are usually reserved for patients who fail with other oral regimens; most common with chronic azole administration and azole-resistant *Candida* species

In vitro resistance is most common with prior azole exposure, late stage HIV infection, and non-albicans species. Some report high rates of response (48/50) to fluconazole despite in vitro resistance (JID 174:821, 1996). Doses up to 800 mg/d may be tried. Alternatives are oral amphotericin and itraconazole 200 mg bid

| Maintenance (optional or as needed: see "Comments") | Clotrimazole (above dose) Fluconazole 100 mg/d po or 200 mg 3×/wk | Itraconazole‡ 200 mg (tabs)/day or 100 mg po suspension qd Ketoconazole‡ 200 mg/d po Nystatin (above dose) | Advantage of fluconazole for maintenance is prevention of deep fungal infection, cryptococcosis, and Candida esophagitis with CD4 count <100/mm^3 (NEJM 332:700, 1995) and reduction of frequent relapses of thrush

Concerns with continuous treatment with fluconazole are azole resistance by Candida species, drug interactions, and cost. Risks for azole resistant Candida infections are prolonged azole exposure and low CD4 count (JID 173:219, 1996)

Fluconazole is superior to clotrimazole in preventing relapses of thrush but risks azole resistance

Most patients will relapse within 3 mo after therapy if treatment is discontinued in absence of immune reconstitution. Options are treatment of each episode or maintenance |

Table 36. (continued)

	Preferred Regimen(s)	Alternative Regimen(s)	Comments
FUNGAL INFECTIONS			
Candida prophylaxis	Not recommended		
Candida vaginitis	Intravaginal miconazole suppository 200 mg × 3 days or cream (2%) × 7 days Clotrimazole cream (1%) × 7–14 days or tabs: 100 mg qd × 7 days or 100 mg × 2/d × 3 days or 500 mg × 1 Fluconazole 150 mg po × 1	Ketoconazole‡ 200 mg/d po or bid × 5–7 days or 200 mg po bid × 3 days	May require continuous treatment to prevent relapse: Ketoconazole 100 mg/d po, fluconazole 50–100 mg/d po, or fluconazole 200 mg/wk po Clotrimazole and miconazole (both cream and 100 mg tabs) are available over-the-counter Weekly fluconazole (200 mg) appears to be effective without risk of azole resistance in women with CD4 count >300/mm³ (Ann Intern Med 1997;126:689) Treatment is identical with and without HIV infection (MMWR 47(RR-1):78, 1998)
Candida esophagitis Initial infection	Fluconazole 200 mg/d po; up to 400 mg/d × 2–3 wk	Itraconazole‡ 100–200 mg po or 100–200 mg oral suspension/day Amphotericin B 0.3–0.5 mg/kg/d IV ± 5-FC 100 mg/kg/d × 5–7 days	Fluconazole is clinically superior to ketoconazole as initial treatment Relapse rate is 84% within 1 yr in absence of prophylaxis after therapy Azole-resistant Candida esophagitis is unusual (CID 30:749, 2000)

Candida Maintenance	Fluconazole 100–200 mg/d po	Ketoconazole 200 mg/d po Itraconazole 200 mg/d po (tabs) or 100 mg/d oral solution	Consider maintenance therapy in all patients with recurrent esophagitis, although probability of resistance is increased (JID 173:219, 1996)
Cryptococcal meningitis Initial treatment (CID 2000; 30:710)	Amphotericin B 0.7 mg/kg/d IV + flucytosine 100 mg/kg/d po × 14 days, then fluconazole 400 mg/d × 8–10 wk *Management of intracraneal pressure:* 1. Focal CNS signs or obtunded—MRI or CT scan before LP, which may show contraindication to LP 2. Normal OP—medical management and LP at 2 wk for culture etc 3. OP >250 mmH₂O—CSF drainage until pressure <200 or 50% initial value; repeat LP daily until nil 4. Elevated pressure persists—lumbar drain or VP shunt	Fluconazole 400 mg/d po × 6–10 wk Itraconazole‡ 200 mg po tid × 3 days, then 200 mg po bid (see "Comments") Fluconazole 400 mg/d po plus flucytosine 100 mg/kg/d po Amphotericin B 0.7 mg/kg/d IV × 14 days (without flucytosine) Ambisome 4 mg/kg/d IV × 14 d	Amphotericin B is preferred for initial treatment, but total dose before fluconazole maintenance is arbitrary Usual tactic is to change to oral fluconazole at 14 days or to make this decision based on CSF cultures at 10–14 days Fluconazole is acceptable as initial treatment only for patients with normal mental status. Other favorable prognostic findings are cryptococcal antigen <1:32 and CSF WBC >20/mm³ Cryptococcal antigen is nearly always detected in CSF and is somewhat useful in monitoring response; sensitivity of **serum** antigen is 99%, usually at titer >1:2048, but it is useless in monitoring response **Itraconazole:** ACTG 159 showed itraconazole (400 mg/d) was as effective as fluconazole (400 mg/d) with 8 wk treatment after initial treatment with amphotericin B 0.7 mg/kg/d ± flucytosine × 14 days (NEJM 337:15, 1997)

Table 36. (continued)

	Preferred Regimen(s)	Alternative Regimen(s)	Comments
FUNGAL INFECTIONS			
			Fluconazole may be used in doses up to 800 mg/d for salvage therapy **5-FC:** Flucytosine + amphotericin B are superior to amphotericin B alone (NEJM 337:15, 1997); flucytosine + fluconazole are also superior to fluconazole alone but show high rates of reactions (CID 26:1362, 1998; CID 19:74, 1994)
Maintenance	Fluconazole 200 mg/d po	Amphotericin B 0.6–1 mg/kg 1–3 ×/wk Fluconazole: May increase maintenance dose to 400 mg/d Itraconazole‡ 200 mg bid	Life-long maintenance treatment required; immune reconstitution may change this recommendation; initial experience is promising but limited Itraconazole in dose of 200 mg/d is inadequate (ICAAC 9/95, abstract 1218); trial with 400 mg/d is ongoing Fluconazole maintenance at 200 mg/d is superior to amphotericin B (NEJM 326:793, 1992) and superior to itraconazole at 200 mg po/d (CID 28:291, 1999)
Prophylaxis (see "Comments")	Not generally recommended	Fluconazole 200 mg po/d Itraconazole 200 mg/po/d or 100 mg oral suspension/d	**Indications:** Consider with high risk patients—those who work with soil and have CD4 count <100/mm³ (JID 179:449, 1999) Efficacy has been shown for all patients with CD4 counts <50/mm³, but concerns are that *Cryptococcus* is infrequent (8–10%), possible azole-resistant *Candida*, possible drug interactions, and cost

Cryptococcosis without meningitis (pulmonary, disseminated, or antigenemia)	Fluconazole 200 mg po bid Indefinitely unless immune reconstitution	Cost analysis is $213,000/quality year of life saved (JAMA 279:13, 1998) All patients with cryptococcosis should have lumbar puncture to exclude meningitis Antigenemia: Chest x-ray, LP, urine and blood culture. If no focus identified and antigenemia persists treat with fluconazole (CID 23:827, 1996)
	Itraconazole‡ 200 mg po bid or 100 mg oral suspension/day	
Maintenance (see "Comments")	Fluconazole 200 mg/d po	Need for maintenance treatment is not established
Histoplasmosis Disseminated, initial treatment	Amphotericin B 0.5–1.0 mg/kg/d IV ≥ 7–14 days Itraconazole‡ 300 mg po bid × 3 days, then 200 mg po bid or 100–200 mg oral suspension bid (mild-moderately severe disease)	Itraconazole‡ 200 mg/d or 100 mg oral suspension/d Amphotericin B 0.6–1 mg/kg IV weekly or 2 ×/wk
		Itraconazole may be used for initial treatment of mild to moderate histoplasmosis without CNS involvement or it may be used for maintenance therapy after induction with amphotericin B (Am J Med 98:336, 1995) Should verify itraconazole levels (San Antonio Lab 210-567-4131 or Indianapolis Lab 317-630-2515) Fluconazole is less active than itraconazole and may require doses of 600–800 mg/d for primary or maintenance therapy; ketoconazole is not recommended
	Fluconazole 1600 mg po × 1, then 800 mg/d × 12 wk, then 400 mg/d (Am J Med 103:223, 1997)	
Maintenance	Itraconazole‡ 200 mg po bid	Amphotericin B 1.0 mg/kg 1 ×/wk Fluconazole 400 mg po/d
		Efficacy of itraconazole is established (Ann Intern Med 118:610, 1993) Itraconazole is superior to fluconazole (Am J Med 103:223, 1997) Data are inadequate to provide guidelines for discontinuation of maintenance therapy owing to immune reconstitution

Table 36. (continued)

	Preferred Regimen(s)	Alternative Regimen(s)	Comments
FUNGAL INFECTIONS			
Prophylaxis	Itraconazole‡ 200 mg po/d	Fluconazole 200 mg po/d	**Indication:** Consider in endemic area with CD4 <100/mm³, especially if at high risk owing to occupation (work with soil) or hyperendemic rate (>10 cases/100 patient-yr) (MMWR 48(RR-10):24, 1999)
Coccidioidomycosis Initial treatment	Amphotericin B 0.5 mg/kg/d IV × ≥ 8 wk; total dose 2–2.5 g Fluconazole 400–800 mg po qd Itraconazole‡ 200 mg po bid		Intrathecal amphotericin B usually added for coccidioidomycosis meningitis Fluconazole preferred for meningitis (Ann Intern Med 119:28, 1993)
Maintenance	Fluconazole 400 mg/d Itraconazole‡ 200 mg po bid	Amphotericin B 1 mg/kg/wk	Fluconazole often preferred because of more predictable absorption and fewer drug interactions (Antimicrobial Agents Chemother 39:1907, 1995) Maintenance therapy is life long regardless of immune reconstitution
Prophylaxis			Not recommended
Penicillium marneffei (Penicilliosis)	Amphotericin B 0.7–1.0 mg/kg/d Itraconazole 400 mg po/d		Fever ± pneumonitis, adenopathy, skin, and mucosal lesions (papules, nodules, or pustules) Endemic in Thailand, Hong Kong, China, Vietnam, and Indonesia (Emerg Infect Dis 2:109, 1996; Lancet 344:110, 1994)

			In vitro sensitivity tests show good activity for amphotericin B, ketoconazole, itraconazole, miconazole, and 5FC (J Mycol Med 5:21, 1995; AAC 37:2407, 1993)
Maintenance	Itraconazole 200 mg po/d	Ketoconazole	Lifelong treatment required (NEJM 339:1739, 1998)

PARASITIC INFECTIONS

Toxoplasma gondii **encephalitis** Acute infection	Pyrimethamine 100–200 mg loading dose, then 50–100 mg/d po + folinic acid 10 mg/d po + sulfadiazine or trisulfapyrimidine 4–8 g/d po for at least 6 wk	Pyrimethamine + folinic acid (see preferred regimen) + clindamycin 900–1200* mg IV q6h or 300–450 mg po q6h for at least 6 wk. Pyrimethamine and folinic acid (see preferred regimen) plus one of the following: Azithromycin 1200–1500 mg/d, clarithromycin 1 g bid, or atovaquone 750 mg with food qid. Azithromycin 900 mg po × 2 1st day, then 1200 mg/d × 6 wk, then 600 mg/d (patients <50 kg receive half dose) (salvage therapy). Experimental: Azithromycin, clarithromycin, trimethrexate, doxycycline, atovaquone. Azithromycin for IV use: 500 mg × 2 1st day, then 500 mg/d × 9 days, then oral regimen	Anticipated response is clinical improvement within 1 wk and improvement by CT scan or MRI within 2 wk. Failure to respond and/or uncertain diagnosis is usually an indication for stereotactic brain biopsy, which has excellent diagnostic yield and good safety record (CID 30:49, 2000). Corticosteroids if significant edema/mass effect (Decadron 4 mg po or IV q6h). Pyrimethamine usually given as a loading dose of 200 mg followed by 50 mg. Controlled trial in 340 patients showed pyrimethamine (50 mg/d) plus sulfadiazine (4 g/d × 8 wk, then 2 g/d) was superior to pyrimethamine (50 mg/d) plus clindamycin (2.4 g/d × 8 wk, then 1.2 g/d) (CID 22:268, 1996)

Table 36. (continued)

	Preferred Regimen(s)	Alternative Regimen(s)	Comments
		PARASITIC INFECTIONS	
T. gondii encephalitis Suppressive therapy	Pyrimethamine 25–75 mg po qd + folinic acid 10 mg qd + sulfadiazine 0.5–1.0 g po qid	Pyrimethamine 25–75 mg/d po + folinic acid 10–25 mg qd + clindamycin 300–450 mg po q 6–8 hr Alternatives without established efficacy: Pyrimethamine 25–75 mg/d po + folinic acid 10–25 mg qd + either atovaquone 750 mg q8–12h, dapsone* 100 mg/d po, or azithromycin 600 mg/d po	Regimens with established efficacy are pyrimethamine plus sulfonamide or clindamycin Pyrimethamine-sulfadiazine, TMP-SMX, and atovaquone ± pyrimethamine provide *P. carinii* prophylaxis; pyrimethamine-clindamycin does not Treatment is lifelong unless there is immune reconstitution (see below)
T. gondii encephalitis Prophylaxis (see "Comments")	Trimethoprim-sulfamethoxazole 1 DS po qd	TMP-SMX 1 SS po/d or 1 DS 3 ×/wk Dapsone* 50 mg/d + pyrimethamine 50 mg/wk + folinic acid 25 mg/wk Atovaquone 1500 mg qd ± pyrimethamine 25 mg qd and leucovorin 10 mg qd	**Indications:** Patients with positive toxoplasmosis IgG serology plus CD4 count nadir of <100/mm³. Primary prophylaxis may be discontinued when CD4 count increases to >200/mm³ for >3 mo (Lancet 355:2217; 2000; JID 181:1635, 2000: AIDS 13:1647, 1999) Secondary prophylaxis may be discontinued when CD4 increases to >100–200/mm³ for 6–12 mo (AIDS 13:1647, 1999; AIDS 14:383, 2000) Efficacy for prophylaxis is established for TMP-SMX and dapsone + pyrimethamine and atovaquone ± pyrimethamine. Possibly effective are azithromycin, clarithromycin, Fansidar

Cryptosporidium (Clin Microbiol Rev 12:554; 1999; CID 32:331, 2001)	Paromomycin 500 mg po tid or 1000 mg po bid with food × 14-28 days, then 500 mg po bid Paromomycin 1 g bid + azithromycin 600 mg qd × 4 wk, then paromomycin alone × 8 wk Symptomatic treatment with supplements and antidiarrheal agents: Lomotil, loperamide, paregoric, bismuth subsalicylate (Pepto-Bismol) HAART	Azithromycin 1200 mg × 2 po 1st day, then 1200 mg/d × 27 days, then 600 mg/d, or clarithromycin 500 mg po bid Atovaquone 750 mg po suspension with meal bid Nitazoxanide 500 mg po bid	Efficacy of TMP/SMX at 1 DS qd may be superior to that of lower dose Trials with paromomycin show only modest improvement and no cures (Am J Med 100:370, 1996) Uncontrolled trial of paromomycin plus azithromycin showed good response in terms of clinical symptoms and oocyst excretion (JID 178:900, 1998). Azithromycin alone is ineffective Nitazoxanide (Unimed Pharmaceuticals, Buffalo Grove, IL) is not FDA approved. In ACTG 192 about 30% responded. Usual dose is 500 mg po bid and may be increased to 2000 mg/d HAART with immune reconstitution is most effective treatment (Lancet 351:256, 1998; AIDS 12:35, 1998) Nonsteroidal anti-inflammatory agents are sometimes useful Nutritional supplements often required for severe cases; Vivonex TEN or parenteral hyperalimentation Clarithromycin or rifabutin prophylaxis for MAC prophylaxis may reduce risk of cryptosporidiosis (JAMA 279:384, 1998)

Table 36. (continued)

	Preferred Regimen(s)	Alternative Regimen(s)	Comments
		PARASITIC INFECTIONS	
Isospora Acute infection (CID 32:331, 2001; NEJM 320:1044, 1989)	Trimethoprim + sulfamethoxazole po bid (2 DS po bid or 1 DS tid) × 2–4 wk	Pyrimethamine 50–75 mg/d po + folinic acid 5–10 mg/d × 1 mo	Duration of high-dose therapy is not well defined One case report of refractory infection responded to pyrimethamine plus sulfadiazine (Diagn Microbiol Infect Dis 26:87, 1996)
Suppressive treatment	Trimethoprim + sulfamethoxazole 1–2 DS/ d or 3 × /wk	Pyrimethamine 25 mg + sulfadoxine 500 mg po q wk (1 Fansidar/wk) Pyrimethamine 25 mg + folinic acid 5 mg/d	Treat indefinitely unless there is immune reconstitution
Microsporidiosis (CID 32:331, 2001)	Symptomatic treatment with nutritional supplements and anti-diarrheal agents (Lomotil, Loperamide, paregoric, etc) Albendazole 400 mg po bid × ≥ 3 wk (*S. intestinalis*)	Metronidazole 500 mg po tid Atovaquone 750 mg po tid with meals bid (AIDS 10:619, 1996) Thalidomide 100 mg q d (AIDS 9: 658, 1995)	Efficacy of albendazole is established only for infections involving *Septata intestinalis,* which cause 10–20% of cases Anecdotal success with itraconazole, atovaquone, fluconazole, and metronidazole (Infect Dis Clin North Am 8:483, 1994) HAART with immune reconstitution is the best therapy, especially for the 80–90% of cases involving *E. bieneusi* (Lancet 351:256, 1998; J AIDS 25:124, 2000)

Table 36. (continued) Tuberculosis Treatment Recommendations (MMWR 1998;47[RR-20])

Induction	Maintenance	Comments
RIFAMPIN-BASED THERAPY (NO CONCURRENT USE OF PIS OR NNRTIs)		
1. INH/RIF/PZA/EMB (or SM) daily × 2 mo	INH/R IF daily or 2–3×/wk × 18 wk	Rif-containing regimens preclude concurrent use of protease inhibitors and NNRTI
2. INH/RIF/PZA/EMB (or SM) daily × 2 wk, then 2–3×/wk × 6 wk	INH/RIF or 2–3×/wk × 18 wk	Assess HIV at 3-mo intervals to determine need for antiretroviral therapy
3. INH/RIF/PZA/EMB (or SM) 3×/wk × 8 wk	INH/RIF/PZA/EMB (or SM) 3×/wk × 4 mo	A 2-wk wash-out is required between last RIF dose and initiation of PI or NNRTIs
RIFABUTIN-BASED THERAPY (CONCURRENT PI OR NNRTI)		
1. INH/RFB/PZA/EMB daily × 8 wk	INH/RFB daily or 2×/wk × 18 wk	Monitor for RFB toxicity—arthralgias, uveitis, leukopenia
2. INH/RFB/PZA/EMB daily × 2 wk, then 2×/wk × 6 wk	INH/RFB 2×/wk × 18 wk	Dose modifications of RFB and PIs/NNIRTI when given concurrently (see p 134) RFB should not be given with Invirase, RTV, or DLV
STREPTOMYCIN-BASED THERAPY (CONCURRENT PI OR NNRTI)		
1. INH/SM/PZA/EMB daily × 8 wk	INH/SM/PZA 2–3×/wk × 30 wk	SM is contraindicated in pregnant women
2. INH/SM/PZA/EMB daily × 2 wk, then 2–3×/wk 6 wk	INH/SM/PZA 2–3×/wk × 30 wk	If SM cannot be continued for 9 mo add EMB, and treatment should be extended to 12 mo

INH, isoniazid; RIF, rifampin; RFB, rifabutin; EMB, ethambutol; PZA, pyrazinamide; SM, streptomycin; IDV, indinavir; NFV, nelfinavir; EFV, efavirenz; APV, amprenavir.

Table 36. (continued)
Directly Observed Therapy Two to Three Times Per Week Preferred
(MMWR (47:RR-20), 1998)

	Daily	2×/wk	3×/wk
Isoniazide (INH)	5 mg/kg (300 mg)*	15 mg/kg (900 mg)*	15 mg/kg (900 mg)*
Rifampin*** (RIF)	10 mg/kg (600 mg)*	10 mg/kg (600 mg)*	10 mg/kg (600 mg)*
Rifabutin (RFB)	150–450 mg**	300–450 mg**	300–450 mg**
Pyrazinamide (PZA)	15–30 mg/kg (2 g)*	50–70 mg/kg (4 g)*	50–70 mg/kg (3 g)*
Ethambutol (EMB)	15–25 mg/kg (2.5 g)*	50 mg/kg (2.5 g)*	25–30 mg/kg (2.5 g)*
Streptomycin (SM)	15 mg/kg (1 g)*	25–30 mg/kg (1 g)*	25–30 mg/kg (1 g)*

* Maximum dose.
** Rifabutin (RFB) to be used with antiretroviral regimens including PIs or NNRTIs. See doses below.
*** Rifampin may be used in standard dose with efavirenz, ritonavir, or ritonavir + saquinavir.

TB Treatment Recommendations (continued)
Options for antiretroviral therapy (MMWR 49:183, 2000)
- Regimen that does not contain a protease inhibitor or NNRTI
- Streptomycin-based therapy with no use of rifamycins (see above)
- Rifabutin-based treatment with dose adjustments
- Use rifampin-based regimen with efavirenz, ritonavir, or ritonavir + saquinavir and (?) nevirapine (standard doses for both drugs)

PI or NNRTI	Rifabutin
Indinavir 1000 mg q8h	150 mg/d or 300 mg 2×/wk
Nelfinavir 1000 mg tid or 1250 mg bid	150 mg/d or 300 mg 2×/wk
Amprenavir 1200 mg bid	150 mg/d or 300 mg 2×/wk
Efavirenz 600 mg qd	450–600 mg/d or 600 mg 2×/wk
Ritonavir/saquinavir 400/400 mg bid	150 mg 2–3×/wk
Nevirapine 200 mg bid	300 mg/d
Lopinavir/ritonavir 400/100 mg bid	150 mg qod
Ritonavir 600 mg bid	150 mg qod

No data: Nevirapine and Fortovase; contraindicated: Invirase, delavirdine.

Table 36. (continued)

	Preferred Regimen(s)	Alternative Regimen(s)	Comments
TB prophylaxis INH-susceptible strain (MMWR 49(RR-6), 2000)	Rifampin 600 mg/d + PZA 20 mg/kg/d × 2 mo INH 300 mg/d po + pyridoxine 50 mg/d po × 9 mo INH 900 mg 2×/wk + pyridoxine 50 mg 2×/ wk × 9 mo (DOT)	Rifampin 600 mg po qd × 4 mo plus rifabutin PZA 15–30 mg/kg/d in place of rifampin to permit concurrent PI or NNRTI × 2 mo (see p 134)	**Indications:** PPD ≥5 mm induration, high-risk exposure, or prior positive PPD without treatment CDC preferred regimen is rifampin + pyrazinamide for patients not receiving HAART. Anecdotal cases of 2–3 deaths possibly related—recommendation is to monitor CBC and LFTs at baseline and at week 2, 4 & 6. With HAART: INH regimen × 9 (MMWR 49(RR-6), 2000)
INH-resistant strain	Rifampin 600 mg/d po + pyrazinamide 20 mg/kg × 2 mo	Rifabutin 150–450 mg/d (dose based on concurrent PI or NNRTI) + pyrazinamide × 2 mo Rifabutin × 4 mo	Choice of rifampin vs rifabutin depends on concurrent HAART
Multiply resistant strain	Fluoroquinolone + pyrazinamide or ethambutol + pyrazinamide		Base decision on susceptibility tests and consultation with public health officials
Paradoxical worsening with HAART or immune recovery TB	Antituberculosis drugs + antiinflammatory drugs		Characterized by fever, lymphadenopathy, and pleural effusion usually several weeks after HAART. AFB stains and cultures are often negative (Am J Respir Crit Care Med 158:157, 1998; Am J Med 106:371, 1999; CID 26:1008, 1998)

Table 36. (continued)

	Preferred Regimen(s)	Alternative Regimen(s)	Comments
Mycobacterium avium complex (MAC) bacteremia Treatment	Clarithromycin 500 mg po bid plus ethambutol 15 mg/ kg/d po	Azithromycin 600 mg/d po + ethambutol ± rifabutin in place of clarithromycin + one or more of the drugs listed under "Preferred Regimen(s)" Combination treatment with amikacin 10–15 mg/kg/d IV or ciprofloxacin 500–750 mg bid	Duration is indefinite in absence of immune reconstitution. With HAART, initial results suggest MAC treatment may be discontinued when MAC treatment is >1 yr, CD4 count is >100/mm³ for 3–6 mo, and patient is asymptomatic (JID 178: 1446, 1998) Clarithromycin levels are increased 50–80% with concurrent administration of indinavir, ritonavir, and saquinavir; nelfinavir and amprenavir have no effect on clarithromycin levels In vitro susceptibility tests are not useful in previously untreated patients (CID 27: 1369, 1998) In a comparative trial of azithromycin vs clarithromycin for MAC bacteremia clarithromycin was superior in time to negative blood cultures (CID 27:1278, 1998); another trial showed these macrolides (+ ethambutol) were comparable (CID 31:1254, 2000) Rifabutin dose adjustments with concurrent PIs or NNRTIs: See p 134

| MAC prophylaxis: Initiation and discontinuation | Clarithromycin 500 mg po bid
Azithromycin 1200 mg q wk | Rifabutin 300 mg/po qd (adjust dose if given with PI or NNRTI)
Azithromycin 1200 mg qd plus rifabutin 300 mg po qd | Drug interaction between clarithromycin and rifabutin results in decreased levels of clarithromycin (NEJM 335:428, 1996; JID 181:1289, 2000)
ASA or NSAID often effective for symptom relief
Clarithromycin at a dose >1000 mg/d was associated with increased mortality (Ann Intern Med 121:905, 1994)

Indications: <50/mm^3
Discontinuation: Primary prophylaxis may be discontinued in patients who respond to HAART with increases in CD4 counts to >100/mm^3 for ≥3 mo (NEJM 335:392, 1996; Lancet 355:2217, 2000; JID 181:1635, 2000)
Patients who have had disseminated MAC may discontinue secondary prophylaxis when treated ≥1 yr, and the CD4 count is >100–200 for 6–12 mo (AIDS 13:1647, 1999; AIDS 14:383, 2000; JID 178:1446, 1998)
• Preliminary data suggest low dose clarithromycin (500 mg/d) is as effective as 1 g/d (AIDS 13:1367, 1999)
• Azithromycin may contribute to efficacy of PCP prophylaxis with TMP-SMX (Lancet 354:891, 1999)
Prophylaxis failures with clarithromycin or azithromycin often involve clarithromycin-resistant strains |

Table 36. (continued)

	Preferred Regimen(s)	Alternative Regimen(s)	Comments
MAC immune recovery lymphadenitis	Treat for MAC—clarithromycin 500 mg bid + ethambutol 15 mg/kg/d ± anti-inflammatory agents including corticosteroids	Azithromycin + ethambutol Corticosteroids with rapid taper for severe symptoms	Characterized by high fever leukocytosis and lymphadenopathy often involving the periaortic and mesenteric nodes. Less common presentations: bursitis, osteomyelitis, skin nodules, adrenal insufficiency. Biopsy shows granulomatous lymphadenitis with AFB in large numbers. Occurs within 1–3 mo of HAART (Lancet 351:252, 1998; J AIDS 20:122, 1999; Ann Intern Med 133:447, 2000) May require surgical drainage
Mycobacterium kansasii	INH 300 mg po/d + rifampin 600 mg/d po + ethambutol 15–25 mg/kg/d po × 18 mo and for at least 15 mo after sputum conversion ± streptomycin 1 g IM 2×/wk × 3 mo	Also consider ciprofloxacin 750 mg po bid and clarithromycin 500 mg po bid	Experience in HIV-infected patients is limited (J AIDS 4:516, 1991; Ann Intern Med 114: 861, 1991)
Mycobacterium haemophilum	Clarithromycin + ciprofloxacin + rifabutin + amikacin	Cycloserine is active in vitro	Experience is limited (Eur J Clin Microbiol Infect Dis 12:114, 1993)

Mycobacterium gordonae	INH + rifampin + clofazimine or clarithromycin	Streptomycin may be useful	Most isolates are contaminants (Dermatology 187:301, 1993; AIDS 6:1217, 1992; AAC 36:1987, 1992)
Mycobacterium genavense	Clarithromycin + ethambutol + rifampin	Other possible agents: Ciprofloxacin and pyrazinamide	Clarithromycin-containing regimens are most effective (AIDS 7:1357, 1993)
Mycobacterium xenopi	INH/rifampin/ ethambutol/ streptomycin		
Mycobacterium malmoense	Rifampin/INH/ ethambutol		CID 16:540, 1993
Mycobacterium chelonei	Clarithromycin 500 mg bid × ≥6 mo	Variable activity: Cefoxitin, amikacin, doxycycline, imipenem, tobramycin	Need in vitro sensitivity tests
Mycobacterium fortuitum	Amikacin 400 mg IV q12h + cefoxitin 12 g IV/d × 2–4 wk, then oral agents based on in vitro sensitivity tests		Usual oral agents—clarithromycin, doxycycline, sulfamethoxazole, ciprofloxacin

VIRUSES

Herpes simplex Initial treatment mild	Acyclovir 400 mg po 3×/day or famciclovir 250 mg po tid or valacyclovir 1.0 g po bid; all given 7–10 days		Failure to respond: Give valacyclovir or give acyclovir IV

Table 36. (continued)

	Preferred Regimen(s)	Alternative Regimen(s)	Comments
VIRUSES			
Severe or refractory	Acyclovir 15 mg/kg IV/day at least 7 days	Foscarnet 40 mg/kg IV q8h or 60 mg/kg q12h × 3 wk Topical trifluridine as 1% ophthalmic solution q8h	If fails to respond give acyclovir 30 mg/kg/d IV and test sensitivity of isolate to acyclovir; Treatment of resistant HSV: IV foscarnet, topical trifluridine, oral valacyclovir, or high-dose IV acyclovir (12–15 mg/kg IV q8h or by continuous infusion). Relapses after treatment of acyclovir-resistant strains often involve acyclovir-sensitive strains Topical trifluridine solution (Viroptic 1%) is applied after H_2O_2 cleaning and gentle gauze debridement; cover with nonabsorbent gauze with bacitracin and polymyxin ointment
HSV—recurrent	Acyclovir 400 mg po tid or 800 mg po bid or famciclovir 125 mg po bid or valacyclovir 500 mg po bid; all given 5 days		Early treatment is much more effective
HSV—prophylaxis	Acyclovir 400 mg po bid or famciclovir 125–250 mg po bid or valacyclovir 500 mg po qd or bid		Alternative is to treat each episode Patients receiving ganciclovir, foscarnet, or cidofovir do not require acyclovir prophylaxis

			Comments
HSV—visceral	Acyclovir 30 mg/kg IV/day at least 10 days	Foscarnet 40 mg/kg IV q8h × ≥10 days Valacyclovir 1.0 g po tid	
Herpes zoster Dermatomal	Acyclovir 800 mg po 5×/day at least 7 days (until lesions crust) or famciclovir 500 mg po tid or valacyclovir 1 g po tid	Acyclovir 30 mg/kg/d IV Foscarnet 40 mg/kg IV q8h or 60 mg/kg IV q12h	Some authorities recommend corticosteroids (Ann Intern Med 125:376, 1996); prednisone 60 mg × 7 days, 30 mg days 8–14, 15 mg days 15–21 Postherpetic neuralgia is less common in young patients; no maintenance therapy recommended Foscarnet preferred for acyclovir-resistant cases Comparative trial of acyclovir vs valacyclovir showed slight advantage to valacyclovir (AAC 39:1546, 1995) Treatment can be started as long as new lesions are forming
VZV—disseminated, ophthalmic nerve involvement or visceral	Acyclovir 30–36 mg/kg IV/day at least 7 days	Foscarnet 40 mg/kg IV q8h or 60 mg/kg q12h	
VZV—acyclovir-resistant strains	Foscarnet 40 mg/kg IV q8h or 60 mg/kg IV q12h		Role of maintenance therapy unclear
VZV—maintenance (see "Comments")	Acyclovir, famciclovir, or valacyclovir po in above doses		**Indication:** Frequent recurrences

Table 36. (continued)

	Preferred Regimen(s)	Alternative Regimen(s)	Comments
VIRUSES			
VZV—prevention	Varicella zoster immune globulin (ZVIG) 5 vials (6.25 mL) within 96 hr of exposure	Acyclovir 800 mg po 5×/day × 3 wk	**Indication:** Exposure to chickenpox or shingles plus no history of either and, if available, negative VZV serology. Preventive treatment must be initiated within 96 hr of exposure and preferably within 48 hr
Cytomegalovirus retinitis Initial treatment recommendations of the IAS—USA (Arch Intern Med 158:957, 1998; Am J Ophthalmol 127: 329, 1999)	1999 revised IAS guidelines based on HAART related issues: *Patients initiating HAART*—systemic anti-CMV except for Vitrasert for relapse or zone I disease *non-compliant patient*—Vitrasert; *treatment experienced—systemic anti-CMV therapy or Vitrasert; HAART failure*—Vitrasert for zone 1; optional for zones 2 and 3; *systemic therapy* Foscarnet 60 mg/kg IV q8h or 90 mg/kg IV q12h × 14–21 days	Alternating or combining foscarnet and ganciclovir Intraocular injections of foscarnet 1.2–2.4 mg in 0.1 mL (NEJM 330:868, 1994) or ganciclovir 2000 μg in 0.05–0.1 mL (Br J Ophthalmol 1996;80:214) Fomivirsen, 330 μg by intravitreal injection days 1 and 15, then monthly	Median times to progression with initial treatment: Ganciclovir IV 47–104 days, foscarnet IV 53–93 days, ganciclovir + foscarnet IV 129 days, oral ganciclovir 29–53 days, ganciclovir implant (Vitrasert) 216–226 days, cidofovir IV 64–120 days, fomivirsen intravitreal injection 90–110 days Vitrasert should always be combined with systemic therapy (oral ganciclovir or parenteral agent) to prevent systemic CMV disease and protect contralateral eye Oral ganciclovir should not be used as sole induction therapy. Maintenance with oral ganciclovir is nearly as effective as IV ganciclovir but should be avoided with lesions near the optic nerve or fovea (NEJM 333:615, 1995) Foscarnet requires infusion pump, long infusion time, saline hydration Vitrasert was superior to IV ganciclovir in

time to relapse (220 vs 71 days), but there is increased risk of involvement of the other eye and increased risk of extraocular CMV disease (NEJM 337:83, 1997). The same concern applies to fomivirsen injections. Any local therapy should be accompanied by systemic anti-CMV therapy such as oral ganciclovir (NEJM 337:105, 1997). A large trial showed Vitrasert + oral ganciclovir (4.5 g/d) was as effective as IV ganciclovir (NEJM 390: 1063, 1999)

Alternating or combination ganciclovir plus foscarnet appears less toxic and more active vs CMV compared with foscarnet alone (JID 170:189, 1994)

Indications: Maintenance therapy required life-long for retinitis in patients without immune recovery

Discontinuation

Treatment of CMV may be discontinued when the CD4 count is >100–150/mm^3 for 3–6 mo providing there is concurrence by an ophthalmologist (JAMA 282:1633, 1999; CID 28:528, 1999; Ophthalmology 105:1259, 1998; JID 177:1080, 1998; JID 177:1182, 1998; Am J Ophthalmology 126:817, 1998)

Foscarnet maintenance dose is arbitrary; one study showed 120 mg/kg/d was superior to 90 mg/kg/d in survival and time to progression (JID 167:1184, 1993)

Ganciclovir 5 mg/kg IV bid × 14–21 days
Cidofovir 5 mg/kg/wk × 2, then 5 mg/kg q 2 wk plus probenecid 2 g po 3 hr before each dose, 1 g po at 2 and 8 hr after dose
Local therapy: Vitrasert q6mo + ganciclovir 1–1.5 g po tid

Intravitreous injections of fomivirsen, ganciclovir, foscarnet, or cidofovir + oral ganciclovir (Ophthalmology 105:1404, 1998; Ophthalmology 102:533 1995; NEJM 340:1063, 1999)

Maintenance

Foscarnet IV 90–120 mg/kg d
Ganciclovir 5–6 mg/kg/d IV 5–7 d/wk or 1000 mg po tid
Cidofovir 5 mg/kg IV every other week
Vitrasert q 6 mo + oral ganciclovir 1 g po tid

Table 36. (continued)

	Preferred Regimen(s)	Alternative Regimen(s)	Comments
VIRUSES			
			See above for median time to relapse for different initial regimens
Progression (on maintenance therapy)	Vitrasert if not used initially Increase dose of same agent to induction doses (ganciclovir 10 mg/kg/d or foscarnet 120 mg/kg/d) **or** switch to alternative drug (induction doses) Combination treatment with ganciclovir + foscarnet in maintenance doses (JID 168:144, 1993; Am J Ophthalmol 117:776, 1994; Arch Ophthalmol 114:23, 1996)	Cidofovir 5 mg/kg (as above) Fomivirsen 330 µg by intravitreal injection days 1 and 15, then monthly Cidofovir (as above) + ganciclovir 1 g po tid with meal	Time to relapse varies with definition; and treatment as summarized above. Subsequent relapses occur more rapidly ACTG 228 showed no difference between reinduction with the same drug compared with switching to alternative drug. With combination treatment, there was the best outcome for time to progression (4.8 mo vs 1.6–2.1 mo) and the worst for quality of life (presumably because of time required for infusions) (Arch Ophthalmol 114:23, 1996) Preliminary data for cidofovir + oral ganciclovir show good response rates and good anti-CMV effect, but high rates of drug-related toxicity (CID 28:528, 1999) If ganciclovir implant fails consider IV or intravitreal foscarnet owing to possible ganciclovir resistance

Immune recovery vitritis	Systemic or periocular corticosteroids		Posterior segment inflammation in patients with inactive CMV retinitis and immune recovery associated with HAART (Arch Ophthalmol 116:169, 1998) Incidence is highly variable for reasons that are unclear—up to 40% in some series (JAMA 283:653, 2000; Ann Intern Med 133:447, 2000; JID 179:697, 1999) Must exclude other causes of uveitis including TB, syphilis, toxoplasmosis, lymphoma, and drug reactions (Am J Ophthalmol 125:292, 1998)
Cytomegalovirus extra-ocular disease Gastrointestinal	Ganciclovir 5 mg/kg IV bid × 3–6 wk Foscarnet 60 mg/kg q8h or 90 mg/kg IV q12h × 3–6 wk	Failure: Ganciclovir + foscarnet	Ganciclovir and foscarnet are equally effective for CMV colitis (Am J Gastroenterol 88:542, 1993) Maintenance therapy should be considered, especially after re-induction and relapse; discontinuation of maintenance should be considered when CD4 count is >100–150/mm^3 × 3–6 mo Role of oral ganciclovir is unclear Patients should have regular ophthalmoscopic screening Foscarnet plus ganciclovir are associated with poor quality of life (JID 167:1184, 1993)
Neurologic disease	As above or ganciclovir + foscarnet		Combination therapy with ganciclovir + foscarnet is probably optimal, but quality of life is poor and prognosis with any form of therapy (except possibly HAART) is also poor. Median survival in the HAART era is reported at 3 mo (AIDS 14:517, 2000)

Table 36. (continued)

	Preferred Regimen(s)	Alternative Regimen(s)	Comments
		VIRUSES	
			Cidofovir: Experience is nil with neurologic disease
			Treatment does not extend survival, and irreversible damage is often present when treatment is started (Neurology 46:444, 1996)
			Maintenance therapy should be given after induction phase and can presumably be considered for discontinuation when CD4 count is >100–150/mm^3 × 3–6 mo
Pneumonia	Ganciclovir 5 mg/kg IV bid ≥21 days Foscarnet 60 mg/kg q8h or 90 mg/kg IV q12h ≥21 days		Minimum diagnostic criteria: 1) Pulmonary infiltrates; 2) detection of CMV with culture antigen or nucleic acid studies of pulmonary secretions; 3) characteristic intracellular inclusions in lung tissue or BAL macrophages; and 4) absence of another pulmonary pathogen (Arch Intern Med 158:957, 1998)
			Consider therapy if there is a copathogen that fails to respond to therapy
			Long-term maintenance therapy is usually unnecessary unless there is relapse or extra-pulmonary end organ disease

Progressive multifocal leukoencephalopathy (PML)	Highly active antiretroviral regimen (HAART)	Multiple studies suggest potential utility of HAART, but results are inconsistent (AIDS 13:1881, 1999; CID 28:1152, 1999; CID 30: 95, 2000). Largest series with 57 patients given HAART showed improvement in 26% and development of new lesions in 16% (JID 182:1077, 2000)
	Cidofovir (?)	

BACTERIA

Streptococcus pneumoniae Treatment	Penicillin, amoxicillin, cefotaxime, ceftriaxone (see "Comments")	Rates of resistance are increasing as indicated by the CDC report of 3475 strains from invasive pneumococcal infections in 1998 (NEJM 343:1917, 2000). These studies show the following rates of resistance: Penicillin—14%, cefotaxime—6%, macrolides—11%, clindamycin—4%, tetracycline—6%, TMP-SMX—23%, fluoroquinolones—0.5%, vancomycin—0%
	Macrolide, vancomycin, levofloxacin, gatifloxacin, moxifloxacin	Strains highly resistant to penicillin should be treated with vancomycin or newer quinolones (levofloxacin, moxifloxacin, gatifloxacin). TMP-SMX is now considered inadequate for empiric use owing to high rates of resistance
Prevention	CD4 count >200/mm³; Pneumococcal vaccine 0.5 mL SC	Repeat at 5-yr intervals or at time of immune recovery with CD4 >200 if initial vaccination was performed when CD4 count was <200/mm³
	None	Response with CD4 count <200/mm³ is limited

Table 36. (continued)

	Preferred Regimen(s)	Alternative Regimen(s)	Comments
		BACTERIA	
Haemophilus influenzae	Cefuroxime	TMP-SMX Cephalosporins, 2nd and 3rd generation Fluoroquinolones	Traditional therapy usually adequate (CID 30:461, 2000) *H. influenzae* vaccine is not recommended for adults because most infections involve nonencapsulated strains
Nocardia asteroides	Sulfadiazine or trisulfapyridine 4–8 g po or IV/day to maintain sulfa level at 15–20 μg/mL	Trimethoprim-sulfa 4–6 DS/day Minocycline 100 mg po bid Other suggested regimens: Imipenem + amikacin; sulfonamide + amikacin or minocycline; ceftriaxone + amikacin	
Pseudomonas aeruginosa	Aminoglycoside + antipseudomonal beta-lactam (ticarcillin, piperacillin, mezlocillin, ceftazidime, cefepime), imipenem, or ciprofloxacin	Monotherapy with an antipseudomonal beta-lactam (ceftazidime or cefoperazone, cefepime), ciprofloxacin, or imipenem/meropenem	Antibiotic selection requires in vitro susceptibility data. Need for "double coverage" is disputed
Rhodococcus equi	Vancomycin 2 g/d IV ± rifampin 600 mg po qd, ciprofloxacin 750 mg po bid or imipenem 0.5 g IV qid × 2–4 wk	Erythromycin 2–4 g/d IV	Ciprofloxacin 750 mg po bid may be used for long-term maintenance, but resistance is likely to develop Also sensitive to rifampin and aminoglycosides; resistant in vitro to penicillins and cephalosporins

Organism			
Bartonella henselae/quintana (bacillary angiomatosis)	Erythromycin 250–500 mg po qid × ≥8 wk or doxycycline 100 mg po bid ≥8 wk	Other macrolides	Macrolide for MAC prophylaxis is protective. May require life-long therapy
Salmonella Acute (CID 32:331, 2001)	Ciprofloxacin 500 mg po bid × ≥2 wk. Ofloxacin 300 mg po bid × ≥2 wk	Trimethoprim 5–10 mg/kg/d + sulfamethoxazole IV or 1 DS bid × ≥2 wk (preferred if sensitive). Cephalosporins; 3rd generation	Relapse is common. Eradication of *Salmonella* has been demonstrated only for ciprofloxacin. AZT is active vs most *Salmonella* strains and may be effective prophylaxis. Drug selection requires in vitro susceptibility data especially for ampicillin. Recommendations are based on 1 DSA guidelines (CID 32:331, 2001)
Maintenance	Ciprofloxacin 500 mg po bid × several mo	Trimethoprim-sulfamethoxazole 5 mg/kg/d, trimethoprim (1 DS po bid)	Indications for maintenance therapy, specific regimens, and duration not well defined
Staphylococcus aureus	Antistaphylococcal penicillin (nafcillin, oxacillin) or cefazolin ± gentamicin 1 mg/kg IV q8h or rifampin 300 mg po bid. Oral agents: Cephalexin 500 mg po qid, dicloxacillin 500 mg po qid, ciprofloxacin 750 mg po qid, or clindamycin 300 mg po qid	Vancomycin 1 g IV bid × 14–28 days ± gentamicin 1 mg/kg IV q8h × 3 days or rifampin 300 mg po bid × 14–28 days. Ciprofloxacin 750 mg po bid + rifampin 300 mg po bid × 28 days	MRSA strains must be treated with vancomycin or linezolid. Use of ciprofloxacin or other quinolone requires in vitro sensitivity tests. Regimen and duration depend on site of infection and in vitro sensitivity tests. Fluoroquinolone regimen requires demonstration of in vitro activity. Duration of therapy is arbitrary; 2-wk regimen appears adequate for most

Table 36. (continued)

	Preferred Regimen(s)	Alternative Regimen(s)	Comments
		BACTERIA	
	Tricuspid valve endocarditis: Nafcillin or oxacillin 3 g IV q6h × 14–28 days + gentamicin 1.0 mg/kg IV q8h × 3 days		
Treponema pallidum (MMWR 47(RR-1):38, 1998)	Primary secondary syphilis and early latent (<1 yr): Benzathine penicillin G 2.4 mil units IM weekly × 1 (see "Comments") Latent syphilis: Benzathine penicillin G 2.4 mil units IM weekly × 3	No alternative considered adequate for HIV-infected patients; if history of penicillin allergy then perform skin test if reagents available (major and minor)—if positive skin test or positive history and no skin test then desensitize	Follow-up clinically and serologically at 2, 3, 6, 9, and 12 mo Patients with latent syphilis of uncertain duration are considered to have late latent syphilis LP is recommended with neurologic symptoms, treatment failure, and late latent syphilis

Neurosyphilis: Aqueous penicillin G 18–24 mil units/day IV × 10–14 days (3–4 mil units q4h)

Abbreviations:
AMB, amphotericin B

AMP, amprenavir
AZT, zidovudine
Cipro, ciprofloxacin
CMV, cytomegalovirus
CT, computed tomographic scan
DLV, delavirdine
EFV, efavirenz
EMB, ethambutol
5-FC, flucytosine (5-fluorocytosine)
FUO, fever of unknown origin
G-CSF, granulocyte colony-stimulating factor

HAART, highly active anti-retroviral therapy
IDV, indinavir
INH, isoniazid
MRI, magnetic resonance imaging
NFV, nelfinavir
NVP, nevirapine
Oflox, ofloxacin
PCP, *P. carinii* pneumonia
PZA, pyrazinamide
RBT, rifabutin
Rif, rifampin
RTV, ritonavir
SMX, sulfamethoxazole
SQV, saquinavir
Strep, streptomycin
TMP, trimethoprim

* Patients with G-6-PD deficiency are at risk for hemolytic anemia when given oxidant drugs such as dapsone, sulfonamides, and primaquine. Some advocate screening all potential recipients; some restrict screening to persons at greatest risk (African-American men, men of Mediterranean descent, men from India or Far East); some simply observe for evidence of hemolysis, which usually occurs in first several days of treatment and often resolves with continued administration. Patients with the Mediterranean variant are at risk for severe hemolysis.

‡ Ketoconazole and, to a lesser extent, the pill form of itraconazole require gastric acid for absorption; absorption with hypochlorhydria may be enhanced by administration with 0.2 N HCl or the following soft drinks: Coca-Cola, Diet Coke, Pepsi, ginger ale, and Diet Minute Maid orange juice (AAC 39:1671, 1995). Liquid formulation of itraconazole is preferred to capsules for thrush, for patients with achlorhydria, and those with subtherapeutic trough serum levels with capsules (<2 μg/mL); some consider the liquid formulation to be the preferred form for all oral itraconazole therapy, although all clinical trials except for thrush and *Candida* esophagitis were conducted with the capsule form.

Table 37. Treatment of Miscellaneous and Noninfectious Disease Complications Classified by Organ System

Condition	Treatment	Comments
Cardiac Cardiomyopathy J AIDS 18:145, 1998)	Digitalis, diuretic, and cautious use of ACE inhibitors Some patients respond to antiretroviral therapy (HAART) ACE inhibitors, i.e., enalapril 2.5 mg bid titrated to 20 mg/d as tolerated or captopril 6.25 mg tid titrated to 25–50 mg tid May need to add digitals ± diuretics Use of NSAIDS and prednisone is controversial	Echocardiograms show dilated cardiomyopathy in up to 8% of HIV-infected patients (NEJM 339:1093, 1998). Biopsies show most have myocarditis and HIV nucleic acid sequences suggesting a direct effect of HIV; other possibilities are immunologically mediated alterations, other cardiotrophic viruses, or drug toxicity caused by AZT and other NRTIs (Ann Intern Med 116:311, 1992) Subclinical cardiac abnormalities are common and correlate with extent of immune suppression (BMJ 309:1605, 1994; NEJM 339:1153, 1998) Infectious causes: *T. gondii*, TB, *C. neoformans*, CMV
Pulmonary Lymphoid interstitial pneumonitis or non-specific interstitial pneumonitis	HAART Prednisone	Possibly caused by HIV infection of the lung Clinical presentation and x-ray resemble PCP, but CD4 is often 200–500. Many patients respond when inadvertently treated for PCP (Am J Respir Crit Care Med 156:912, 1997) Indications and optimal dose of corticosteroid treatment not established; most initiate this treatment after initial observation shows progression; maintenance prednisone sometimes required

Renal Nephropathy (HIV-associated nephropathy—HIVAN)	Antiretroviral therapy (HAART) Hemodialysis (Am J Kidney Dis 29:549, 1997) Hemodialysis and peritoneal dialysis appear equally effective (Am J Kidney Dis 16:1, 1990) Prednisone 60 mg/d × 2–11 wk, then taper 10 mg/wk × 2–26 wk Alternatives: Cyclosporine or ACE inhibitors (J Ped 119:710, 1991; J Am Soc Nephrol 8: 1140, 1997)	Most common is collapsing focal glomerulosclerosis; presents with nephrosis and rapid course to end-stage renal disease in 1–4 mo (Kidney Int 48: 311, 1995) Must distinguish from 1) heroin-associated acute tubular necrosis (including ATN owing to pentamidine, foscarnet, cidofovir, aminoglycosides) and 2) indinavir-associated nephropathy (responds to drug withdrawal). Features of HIVAN are heavy proteinuria, rapid progression, absence of edema, absence of hypertension, and normal sized kidneys Response to steroids appears to be temporary; regimen in ACTG 271 was prednisone 60 mg/d × 6 wk, then taper 10 mg/wk × 6 wk. Uncontrolled trial of 60 mg/d × 2–11 wk with taper over 2–26 wk showed decrease in creatinine in 17/19 and decreased proteinuria in 12/13 (Am J Med 101:41, 1996); five relapsed and responded to retreatment Response to HAART based on clinical and biopsy data has been reported (Lancet 352:783, 1998)
Neurologic Peripheral neuropathy	Discontinue implicated NRTIs (ddC, d4T, ddI) Nortriptyline 10 mg hs: Increase dose by 10 mg q 5 days to maximum of 75 mg hs or 10–20 mg po tid Ibuprofen 600–800 mg tid Topical: Capsaicin-containing ointments (Zostrix, etc). Lidocaine 20–30% ointment for topical use Alternatives: Phenytoin 200–400 mg/d and carbamazepine 200–400 mg po bid	Other tricyclics commonly used: Amitriptyline, desipramine, or imipramine Capsaicin is usually not well tolerated Mexiletine appeared no better than placebo and was inferior to amitriptyline in ACTG 242 One report of two patients suggests response to HAART (Lancet 352:1906, 1998) Acupuncture: A controlled trial failed to show any benefit (JAMA 280:1590, 1998)

Table 37. (continued)

Condition	Treatment	Comments
	Neurontin (gabapentin); 300–800 mg po tid Nerve growth factor (0.3 μg/kg by self SC injection weekly) showed significant efficacy in ACTG 291 but is not yet commercially available Lamotrigine (Lamictal) for failures with other meds	Nucleosides that cause peripheral neuropathy are ddC, ddl and d4T. Rank order: ddl/d4T/HU > ddl/d4T > d4T > ddl (AIDS 14:273, 2000)
Myopathy	Discontinue AZT × 3 wk. Nonsteroidal antiinflammatory agents Prednisone 40–60 mg/d (severe case, biopsy-proven inflammation)	Indication for treatment is proximal muscle weakness plus elevated creatine kinase. Often unclear if caused by HIV or AZT so D/C AZT and monitor clinical and CPK response
HIV-associated dementia (HAD)	Possible benefit from antiretroviral regimens with agents that penetrate CNS (AZT, d4T, hydroxyurea (+ ddl), ABC, nevirapine; less penetration—efavirenz, ddl, 3TC, indinavir) Anecdotal experience indicates response to HAART	Benefit of AZT at higher dose for mild or moderately severe HAD is established; monitor therapy with neurocognitive tests (Ann Neurol 33:343, 1993) CSF levels of HIV RNA respond to HAART in some but not all; response correlates with baseline CD4 count and plasma HIV RNA levels Penetration across blood brain barrier is good for AZT, d4T, nevirapine, and abacavir; it is modest for efavirenz, ddl, 3TC, indinavir, and amprenavir. Best clinical results achieved with HAART regimens that include IDV, EFV, NFV, and NVP (AIDS 12:357, 1998) HAART: Response with immune reconstitution is variable, but the changes appear less impressive than with other HIV-associated complications (AIDS 13:1249, 1999; AIDS 15:195, 2001)

Hematologic *Idiopathic thrombocytopenic purpura (ITP)* Asymptomatic	Antiretroviral regimens that include AZT Discontinue any drugs potentially responsible	Note: Standard treatments (prednisone, IVIG, splenectomy, etc) show response rates of 40-90%; main problem is lack of a durable response (CID 21:415, 1995) Response to AZT may be dose-related; usually responds within 2-4 wk. Utility of other nucleoside analogs is unknown Average increase in platelet count with HAART is 38,000/mm^3 (CID 30:504, 2000)
Severe hemorrhage	Packed red cell/platelet transfusions **plus** prednisone 60-100 mg/d or IVIG 1 g/kg on days 1, 2, 14, and then q 2-3 wk	Initial results with HAART show good response (NEJM 341:1239, 1999)
Persistent symptomatic ITP	Discontinue implicated drugs and avoid nonsteroidal antiinflammatory drugs. HAART	
	AZT 600-1200 mg/d (in combination regimen)	Usual AZT dose is 500-600 mg/d; doses of 1000-1200 mg/d are reserved for non-responders; response is noted in 2-4 wk
	Prednisone 30-60 mg/d with rapid taper to 5-10	Prednisone may be complicated by opportunistic infections, especially thrush and herpes and decreased CD4 count; only 10-20% have persistent response
	IVIG 400 mg/kg days 1, 2, 14 then q2-3wk or	IVIG is highly effective in raising platelet count within 4 days but is expensive, and median duration of response is only 3 wk
	WinRho 50 µg/kg IV over 3-5 min, repeat at day 3-4 prn; may need maintenance therapy at 3- to 4-wk intervals using 25-60 µg/kg	WinRho is an alternative to IVIG in Rh-positive ITP patients. Advantages are 3- to 5-min infusions, good safety profile, and reduced cost (Blood 77:1884, 1991)

Table 37. (continued)

Condition	Treatment	Comments
	Splenectomy	Utility with splenectomy is debated: durability of response is variable and some claim risk of HIV progression is increased (Lancet 2:342, 1987); others claim good long-term results (Arch Surg 124:625, 1989)
	Splenic irradiation, danazol, vincristine, interferon	Experimental or experience limited with all four
Anemia	Treatment based on cause HAART	Two causes are 1) decreased production: infiltration tumor (lymphoma, KS), infection (MAC, TB, parvovirus B 19, CMV, histoplasmosis), drugs (AZT, amphotericin, ganciclovir, hydroxyuria, pyrimethamine, interferon), anemia of chronic disease, deficiency status (Fe, vitamin B_{12}, folic acid) or HIV inhibition of precursors (CID 30:405, 2000) 2) Increased destruction (hemolysis) TTP, drugs (sulfonamides, dapsone, primethamine + G6PD deficiency)
	Parvovirus B 19: IVIG	Parvovirus B 19: Marrow shows giant pronormoblasts with clumped basophilic chromatin and clear cytoplasmic vacuoles—diagnosis by in situ hybridization

Anemia algorithm for EPO

EPO candidate: Hct <30%, Hgb <9 g/dL

Exclude bleeding (stool guaiac), hemolysis (smear), and iron deficiency (serum iron, transferin, % saturation, and ferritin)

Underlying cause

Correct

Initiate EPO 40,000 units SC q wk (± supplemental iron)

Monitor response that will usually not be seen for ≥2 wk

Hgb ↑ >1 g/dL at 4 wk: Continue same dose

Hgb increase <1 g/dL at 4 wk: Increase to 60,000 units q wk

Monitor therapy at this dose

Hgb >11–13 g/dL: Hold EPO or decrease by 10,000 units/wk

Hgb increase <1 g/dL at wk 12: Discontinue

Neutropenia

Discontinue drugs that cause neutropenia when posssible

Most likely agents: AZT and ganciclovir; others 3TC, ddI, d4T, foscarnet, ribavirin, flucytosine, amphotericin, sulfonamide pyrimethamine, pentamidine, antineoplastic agent, and interferon

Reported risk is variable; largest analysis showed higher risk for hospitalization with ANC <500 (Arch Intern Med 157:1825, 1997)

G-CSF (Neupogen) or GM-CSF (Leukine) 1–10 µg/kg/d SC; usual initial dose of G-CSF is 1 µg/kg/d with increases of 1 µg/kg/d at 5- to 7-day intervals to maintain ANC at 1000–2000/mm³; usual maintenance dose is 300 µg given 3–7×/wk

G-CSF therapy. Monitor with CBC and diff 2×/wk and titrate up by 1 µg/kg/d or reduce dose 50% q wk for maintenance to keep ANC >1000–2000/mL. Efficacy of G-CSF is established for elevating neutrophil count (NEJM 317:593, 1987)

Table 37. (continued)

Condition	Treatment	Comments
Thrombotic thrombocytopenic purpura	Prednisone 60–100 mg/d plus plasmapheresis	Concern with GM-CSF is possible increased HIV replication, but this is not substantiated in ≥3 trials. Dose recommendations are similar to those given for G-CSF, but starting dose is 5 µg/kg/d (AIDS 12:1151, 1996)
Tumors **Kaposi's sarcoma** **ACTG classification** (Mayo Clin Proc 70:869, 1995)	General	KS generally responds to HAART. CD4 count response is best predictor (AIDS 14: 971, 987, 2000)
Good prognosis: Lesions confined to skin and/or nodes; CD4 >150, no "B symptoms"	Local therapy Topical liquid nitrogen Intralesional vinblastine (0.01–0.002 mg/lesion) q 2 wk × 3 Radiation (low dose, e.g., 400 rads q wk × 6 wk) Laser Systemic therapy	Restrict to few lesions that are small Restrict to few lesions that may be larger (>1 cm) Skin—well tolerated; oral lesion—mucositis common Best with localized lesions Laser, radiation, or vinblastine injection preferred for oral lesions Liposomal anthracyclines are alternatives to ABV chemotherapy that show comparable clinical efficacy and reduced toxicity (AIDS 10:515, 1996)
Poor prognosis: Lesion associated edema, severe oral KS, visceral KS, CD4 <150, history of opportunistic infection, or "B symptoms"	Liposomal daunorubicin (DaunoXome) 40–60 mg/m² IV q2wk or liposomal doxorubicin (Doxil) × 10–20 m/m² Taxol 100–135 mg/m² q 2–3 wk. Adriamycin, bleomycin, and either vincristine or vinblastine (ABV) or vincristine/vinblastine bleomycin/vinca alkaloids Experimental: Foscarnet (Scand J Infect Dis 26:749, 1994); thalidomide (CID 24:501, 1996); HAART; intralesional B-human chorionic gonadotropin 2000 units per lesion; retinolic acid isomers	Systemic therapy is preferred for patients with widespread skin involvement (>25 lesions), extensive cutaneous KS that is nonresponsive to local treatment, extensive edema, and/or symptomatic visceral organ involvement (especially lung KS) (Lancet 346:26, 1995). Taxol is FDA-approved for KS

	Treatment is often limited by drug intolerance or myelosuppression Response rates better for patients with CD4 count >100/mm³; neutropenia common with AZT: Use G-CSF and/or discontinue AZT HHV-8 is susceptible to foscarnet, ganciclovir, and cidofovir (J Clin Invest 99:2082, 1997); role in therapy is unclear. A retrospective analysis of patients with CMV disease showed foscarnet therapy was associated with a significant delay in progression of KS (JAIDS 20:34, 1999): oral or IV ganciclovir given for CMV retinitis will significantly reduce the frequency of KS (NEJM, 340:1063, 1999)
Non-Hodgkin's lymphoma (NHL)	Regimens containing methotrexate, bleomycin, doxorubicin, cyclophosphamide, adriamycin, vincristine, and corticosteroids ± cranial radiation; standard regimens are CHOP and mBACOD + GM-CSF	Low dose chemotherapy is as effective as standard dose (ACTG 142): methotrexate bleomycin 4 units/m², doxorubicin 25 mg/m², cyclophosphamide 300 mg/m², vincristine 1.4 mg/m², dexamethasone 3 μg/m² + GM-CSF 5 μg/kg for ≥four cycles
CNS lymphoma	CNS lymphoma—cranial radiation ± intrathecal cytosine arabinoside (meningitis) ± chemotherapy	
Dermatologic complications Bacillary angiomatosis	Erythromycin 500 mg po qid × ≥8 wk or other macrolide	Alternative: Doxycycline 100 mg bid × ≥8 wk
Molluscum contagiosum	Cryotherapy, electrosurgery, curettage, topical cantharidin or cidofovir HAART	Cidofovir is effective when given IV or topically (Lancet 353:2042, 1999)

Table 37. (continued)

Condition	Treatment	Comments
Eosinophilic folliculitis	Cetirizine or loratadine + topical steroids Ultraviolet light	Requires constant light Efficacy of UV light established (NEJM 318: 1183, 1988)
Staphylococcal folliculitis	Cephalexin or dicloxacillin 500 mg po qid × 7–21 days	Add rifampin 600 mg/d × 7 days if severe or refractory Recurrent disease: Chronic antibiotic (clindamycin 150 mg q d or TMP-SMX 1 DS q d) and/or nasal mupirocin
Dermatophytic fungi	Skin—topical miconazole or clotrimazole. Refractory cases: Ketoconazole 200 mg po/ day × 1–3 mo or itraconazole 100 mg/d Nails—griseofulvin 660 mg/d × 6–15 mo or itraconazole 200 mg bid × 1 wk/mo × 2 (fingernails) or 3–4 mo (toenails) or terbinafine 250 mg/d × 6 wk (fingernails) or 12 wk (toenails)	Ointments (miconazole and clotrimazole) are over-the-counter
Seborrhea	Skin—steroid cream (hydrocortisone 1%) and/or topical ketoconazole applied bid Scalp—shampoos containing selenium sulfide, zinc pyrithione, ketoconazole, salicylic acid, or coal tar	Use topical hydrocortisone (2.5%) until lesions resolve, then 1% for maintenance
Gastrointestinal Anorexia	Megace 400–800 mg qd	Weight gain is mostly fat. May lower testosterone levels leading to muscle wasting and impotency

Nausea/vomiting	Dronabinol (Marinol) 2.5 mg po bid	Synthetic THC is active ingredient in marijuana. Weight gain is mostly fat
	Compazine 5–10 mg po q6–8h; Tigan 250 mg po q6–8h; Dramamine 50 mg po q6–8h; Ativan 0.025–0.05 mg/kg IV or IM; haloperidol 1–5 mg bid po or IM; ondansetron (Zofran) 0.2 mg/kg IV or IM; dronabinol 2.5 mg po bid	Phenothiazines (Compazine, etc.), haloperidol (Haldol), trimethobenzamide (Tigan), and metoclopramide (Reglan) may cause dystonia Must consider medications as cause of nausea
Pancreatitis	Discontinue any implicated drug NPO ± parenteral hyperalimentation	May be due to adverse drug reaction (especially ddI, d4T, both, or pentamidine), primary HIV infection, or opportunistic infection (CMV, mycobacteria, cryptococcosis) (Am J Med 1995;3:243)
Mouth Aphthous ulcers	Mouth rinses with Mile's solution, dexamethasone (0.5 mg/mL), Dyclone (10%), Benadryl, or viscous lidocaine (2%) Topical fluocinonide (Lidex) 0.05% ointment mixed 1:1 with Orabase	Mile's solution—60 mg hydrocortisone, 20 mL mycostatin, 2 g tetracycline, and 120 mL viscous lidocaine Lesions are considered major or minor on basis of size, depth, and duration. Major lesions are >1 cm deep, usually painful, usually persistent, and often recur
	Thalidomide 100–200 mg/day with increase up to 400–600 mg/d if unresponsive. After healing discontinue or use maintenance dose of 50 mg/d (J Am Acad Dermatol 1993;28:271)	Thalidomide is available from Celegene (888-4235436) which has requirements for physician, patient, and pharmacist. Experience to date is good (NEJM 1997; 337:1086; CID 1995;20:250; JID 1999;180: 61)
	Colchicine 1.5 mg/d (J Am Acad Dermatol 1994;31:459) Intralesional or topical corticosteroids Prednisone 40 mg/d po × 1–2 wk, then taper (severe or refractory cases)	

Table 37. (continued)

Condition	Treatment	Comments
Oral hairy leukoplakia	Acyclovir 800 mg po 5×/day × 2–3 wk	Most relapse and may require maintenance high-dose acyclovir Famciclovir, valacyclovir, foscarnet, ganciclovir shoud be as effective as acyclovir Most lesions are asymptomatic and do not require treatment; relapses are common when acyclovir is discontinued and may require acyclovir maintenance therapy
Salivary gland enlargement	Xerostomia: Sugarless gum and artificial saliva; pilocarpine for refractory cases Painful cystic lesions: Needle aspiration	CT scan will distinguish cystic and solid lesions (Laryngoscope 98:772, 1988). Biopsy if malignancy is suspected (most are benign cystic lesions.) Fine needle aspirate permits microbiologic analysis and decompression
Gingivitis/periodontitis	Curettage and debridement of involved tissue + topical antiseptic such as povidone—iodine solution and chlorhexidine (Peridex) mouth rinses Metronidazole 250 mg tid or 500 mg po bid × 7–14 days or clindamycin 300 mg tid × 7–14 days in selected cases	Four phases: Gingival erythema, necrotizing gingivitis, necrotizing peridontitis, and necrotizing stomatitis (Ann Intern Med 125:485, 1996) Usual presenting complaints are oral pain and bleeding
Esophagitis Candida see p 120		
Cytomegalovirus see p 140		
Herpes simplex see p 137		

Aphthous ulcer

Prednisone 40 mg/d po × 2 wk, then slow taper

Thalidomide 100–200 mg/d, increase to 400–600 prn as tolerated. When needed D/C thalidomide or use maintenance dose of 50 mg/d

Thalidomide is available through the STEPS program (888-423-5436). Concern is teratogenic side effect. Data for response of aphthous ulcers are good (BMJ 289:432, 1989; NEJM 337:1086, 1997; AIDS Res Human Retroviruses 13:301, 1997; CID 20:250, 1995)

Diarrhea
Specific microbial agent
CID 32:331, 2001

C. difficile: Metronidazole 500 mg po tid × 10–14 d
Travelers diarrhea: Ciprofloxacin 500 mg bid × 3 d or TMP-SMX 1 DS bid × 3 d
C. jejuni: Cipro 500 mg bid × 3–5 d; erythro 500 mg po bid × 5 d
Salmonella: Cipro 500 mg bid × 14 d; cefotaxime 4–8 g/d IV × 14 d
Shigella: TMP-SMX 1 DS bid × 7–10 d
Aeromonas: TMP-SMX 1 DS bid × 3 d; cipro 500 mg bid × 3 d
E. histolytica: Metronidazole 750 mg po or IV tid × 5–10 d + paromomycin 500 mg po tid × 7 d
Giardia: Metronidazole 250–750 mg po tid × 7–10 d
Cryptosporidia, Isospora, microsporidia—see p 131–132

Recommendations are IDSA guidelines

Bacterial overgrowth

Doxycycline 100 mg po bid, metronidazole 500–750 mg po bid, or amoxicillin-clavulanate 500 mg po qid

Diagnosis requires quantitative culture of small bowel aspirate or hydrogen breath test

Symptomatic treatment

Lomotil/loperamide/paregoric, etc
Diet modification—low fat, no caffeine, no milk, or milk products

Utility of bismuth salts (Pepto-Bismol) and indomethacin unknown

Table 37. (continued)

Condition	Treatment	Comments
Protease inhibitor associated diarrhea (CID 30:908, 2000)	Loperamide—4 mg, then 2 mg with each loose stool, up to 16/d Psyllium 1 tsp bid or 2 bars qd - bid Oat bran 1500 mg bid Calcium 500 mg bid Fiber supplements Pancreatic supplements, 1-2 tabs with meals	Over-the-counter loperamide, psyllium, oat bran, calcium
Cholangiopathy Papillary stenosis Cholangiopathy without papillary stenosis Isolated duct structure	ERCP with sphincterotomy Ursodeoxycholic acid 300 mg po tid (experience limited) Endoscopic stenting	Presentation: RUQ pain, LFTs show cholestasis; diagnosis established with ERCP. Sensitivity of ultrasound is 75–95% Usual causes are *Cryptosporidium* (most common), microsporidia, CMV, and cyclospora. About 20% are idiopathic Treatment directed against microbial pathogen is unsuccessful for cholangitis Improvement with ursodeoxycholic acid is reported in a small number of patients (Am J Med 103:70, 1997)
Hepatitis C-HIV co-infection	Hepatitis A vaccine if HAV seronegative HCV therapy: Peginterferon 1.5 µg/kg/wk SC (Schering) or 180 µg/wk (Roche) + ribavirin <75 kg – 1000 mg/d: >75 kg – 1200 mg/d × 48 wks	Diagnostic evaluation: see pp 45–46 Indications to treat 47(RR-19), 1998): NIH Consensus (MMWR 1998; 47(RR-19)): 1) Elevated ALT, 2) detectable HCV RNA, and 3) biopsy showing bridging fibrosis or moderate inflammation and necrosis; HCV RNA levels and ALT do not predict prognosis All antiretroviral drugs are potentially hepatotoxic, but chronic HCV infection

does not appear to increase risk of hepatotoxicity (JAMA 2000;283:74).
Ritonavir and nevirapine are probably the most hepatotoxic
Ribavirin can be used with HIV infection, but rate of anemia is high (CID 2000;31:161)
Factors that promote progression of HCV-associated liver disease as HIV co-infection and EtOH abuse
Initial experience with peginterferon is promising (NEJM 2000;343:1666; NEJM 2000;343:1673)

Pancreatitis

Drug associated   D/C implicated drug

Most common—ddI; others—d4T pentamidine, sulfonamides, and corticosteroids; possible causes: INH, 3TC, rifampin, erythromycin, paromomycin

Infection (OIs)   Treat implicated agent

CMV, less common—MAI, TB, cryptosporidium, toxoplasmosis

General causes   Tailor to cause

EtOH, hypertryglyceridemia
ERCP, morbid obesity, cholelithiasis

Wasting
(NEJM 1999;340:1740)

Enteral feedings
Polymeric formulas: Ensure, Sustecal, Enrich, Megnacal, etc

Elemental formulas: Vivonex TEN

Polymeric formulas: Nonprescription about $1.50/can; 10 cans/day required for total caloric needs. Usually not effective in wasting
Elemental diet for severe malabsorption states; often owing to *Cryptosporidium*, microsporidia, or severe CMV infection; parenteral hyperalimentation and feeding gastrostomy rarely used
Parenteral hyperalimentation: Rarely indicated except for devastating diarrhea owing to cryptosporidiosis

Table 37. (continued)

Condition	Treatment	Comments
Pancreatitis Wasting (continued)	Growth hormone (Serostim) 6 mg SC qd × 12 wk	Most weight gain is lean body mass (Ann Intern Med 1996;125:873) Disadvantages are high cost ($1750/wk) need for injection and side effects: Edema, arthralgias, diabetes, pancreatitis, carpal tunnel syndrome May reverse fat redistribution seen with protease inhibitors but concern for ? increased lipoatrophy and glucose intolerance (and cost) Reserve for patients with severe weight loss that is unresponsive to alternative therapy
	Cytokine suppression Thalidomide (Thalomid) 50–300 mg/d × 2–12 wk, usual starting dose is 100 mg/d with increase to 200 mg/d if needed	Thalidomide is available through the STEPS program designed to assure that the men or women do not have that will risk teratogenicity. Call 888-423-5436. Therapeutic trials show good response with weight gain, but high rate of sedation as a side effect (AIDS 1996;10: 1501). Not FDA-approved for this indication
	Appetite stimulants Megace 400–800 mg/d Dronabinol (Marinol) 2.5 mg po bid	Indicated only if weight loss is due to anorexia Megace: Weight gain is mostly fat. May lower testosterone levels with impotence; may cause adrenal insufficiency or diabetes (Ann Intern Med 1994;121:400) Dronabinol: Weight gain is mostly fat

Anabolic steroids

Nandrolone 100–200 mg IM q 1–2 wk

Oxandrolone 20–40 mg/d po (males), 5–20 mg/d po (females)

Testosterone is preferred when there is documented hypogonadism
High anabolic effect and low androgenic effect. Most weight gain is lean body mass (AIDS 1996;10:1657)
Main concern is hepatic toxicity: Peliosis hepatis, cholestatic hepatitis, and hepatic tumors
Safety of nandrolone in women is established by experience with treatment of postmenopausal osteoporosis
Oxandrolone shows highest weight gain of all treatments
May reverse fat redistribution seen with protease inhibitors

Testosterone

Androderm 5 mg/d

Androderm patch 5 mg/d

Testoderm TTS patch 5 mg/d

Testosterone enanthate or testosterone cypionate 200–400 mg IM q 2 wk or 100–200 mg IM q wk by self injection

About 50% of men with AIDS have hypogonadism; benefit is greatest in this group (NEJM 1999;340:1740)
Testosterone is available for oral, injectable, or transdermal use. Oral compounds have been associated with liver toxicity; IM injections consist of an ester in oil that extends half-life to permit weekly or biweekly administration. Transdermal patch is changed daily and worn 22 hr/d. Androderm gel permits graduated changes in dose (Med Lett 2000;42:51)

Serum testosterone levels <450 ng/dL are associated with decreased libido. Drugs associated with decreased testosterone levels are megestrol, ketoconazole, and cimetidine

Table 37. (continued)

Condition	Treatment	Comments
Pancreatitis Wasting (continued)		Testosterone formulations have high androgenic and anabolic effect with improved mood; increased libido, energy, appetite, and lean body mass (CID 1999;28:634)
		May be as effective as growth hormone for fat redistribution with HAART (AIDS 1999;13:1373)
Resistance training	20 min bicycle or treadmill, then 1 hr resistance training 3×/wk	Effective in increasing lean body mass; preliminary results suggest efficacy in fat redistribution syndrome ascribed to protease inhibitors
	Resistance exercise: 20 min/d × 3 days/wk	
Pain (Med Lett 1993;35:1–6)	ASA, acetaminophen, 325–650 mg q4h	Severe pain is best relieved with opioids
	Nosteroidal anti-inflammatory agents (Motrin 200–400 mg q6h; Naprosyn 250–375 q6–8h)	Chronic pain is best treated with nonopioid initially (ASA, acetaminophen, ibuprofen, nortriptyline)
	Codeine 30–60 mg q4–6h po, SC or IM	Dependence liability for opioids
	Meperidine 50–150 mg q3–4h po, SC, IM, IV	Side effects of opioids: Sedation, constipation, respiratory depression, nausea, and vomiting
	Methadone 2.5–10 mg q6–8h po, 10 mg IM	Oral codeine, propoxyphene (Darvon), and pentazocine in usual doses are no more effective than ASA. Morphine, Dilaudid, methadone, levorphanol, fentanyl, and large doses of oxycodone are needed for severe pain
	Dilaudid 2–8 mg q4–8h po or rectal	
	MS Contin 15–60 mg po bid	
	Nortriptyline 25–75 mg qd hs	
	Fentanyl patch 25–100 µg/hr	Morphine and other full agonists have no limit on analgesic effectiveness except for limit ascribed to side effects
	Ultram (tramadol) 50–100 mg q4–6h, up to 400 mg/d	

Psychiatric and sleep disorders

Anxiety	Buspirone (BuSpar) 5 mg tid	Nonbenzodiazepine-nonbarbiturate; dependence liability negligible; increase dose 5 mg q 2–4 days to effective daily dose of 15–30 mg
Depression	Fluoxetine (Prozac) 10 mg increasing to average 20 mg qd	Major side effects are nausea, nervousness, insomnia, weight loss, dry mouth, constipation; insomnia may be treated with Desyrel 25–50 mg hs
	Nortriptyline (Pamelor) 10–25 mg hs increasing to 50–150 mg hs or desipramine (Norpramin) 10–25 mg hs increasing to 50–200 mg hs	Nortriptyline: Titrate level (70–125 mg/dL) promotes sleep. Desipramine (<125 ng/dL) promotes sleep
	Sertraline (Zoloft) 25–50 mg qd increasing to 50–150 mg/d	Side effects are similar to those noted for Prozac but are less severe because of shorter half-life
	Paroxetine (Paxil) 20–50 mg/d po	Promotes sleep; initial dose is 20 mg/d; increase by 10-mg increments
	Bupropion (Wellbutrin) 150 mg bid of SR formulation	Initial dose is 150 mg bid; increase to 300 mg/d after 3 days, as necessary
	Nefazodone (Serzone) 100 mg bid increasing to 300–600 mg/d	Promotes sleep
Delirium	Haldol 0.5–1 mg hs	
Insomnia	Diphenhydramine (Benadryl) 25–50 mg hs	Non-prescription
	Trazodone (Desyrel) 25–100 mg po hs	
	Chloral hydrate 500–1000 mg po hs	Class IV but often considered one of the safest and least habit-forming sedatives
	Ambien 5–10 mg hs	

Table 37. (continued)

Condition	Treatment	Comments
Apathy	Ritalin 7.5 mg bid with weekly increases until intolerance (hyperactivity), adequate response, or maximum dose (60 mg/d) Pemoline 18.75 mg (1 cap) bid with weekly increases to intolerance (shakiness) or response or maximum dose (150 mg/d or 8 caps)	Utility confirmed for both drugs in HIV-infected patients with fatigue associated with depression and psychological distress (Arch Intern Med 161:41, 2001)
Substance abuse	1. Detoxification: Sometimes with long-acting benzodiazepines 2. Treatment of co-morbid conditions: Mental health (depression, bipolar disorder, schizophrenia, personality disorders, etc), medical conditions, and chronic pain syndromes 3. Maintenance treatment and relapse prevention: Individualized to patient need	
Terminal illness	Morphine or other opioids orally or parenterally; MS Contin po 15, 30, 60, or 100 mg; usual dose is 15–60 mg po q12h Patient-controlled analgesia (PCA) for morphine Methadone (above doses) Fentanyl patch	Patients given opioids for acute pain or cancer pain rarely experience euphoria and rarely develop psychic dependence; clinically significant physical dependence develops after several weeks with large doses

9—Drugs Used for HIV-Infected Patients

Table 38. Cost of Drugs Commonly Used in Patients with HIV Infection

Drug	Formulation	Typical Regimen	AWP[a] Unit Price ($)	Cost/Wk ($)	Cost/Yr ($)[b]
Abacavir (Ziagen)	300 mg tabs	300 mg po bid	6.40/300 mg	90	4659
Acyclovir (Zovirax)	200, 400 mg cap	400 mg po bid	2.13/400 mg cap	30	1551
	800 mg tab	800 mg po 4–5×/d	4.10/800 mg tab	140	—
	500 mg vial	2 g/d IV	61.91/500 mg vial	1456	—
Albendazole (Albenza)	200 mg tabs	400–800 mg po bid	1.32/200 mg tab	37–74	—
Alprazolam (Xanax)	0.25, 0.5, 1, and 2 mg tabs	0.25–0.5 mg po bid	0.46/0.25 mg tab	9–18	—
Amikacin (Amikin)	500 mg vial	500 mg bid IV	47.5/1 g vial	840	—
Amoxicillin	250, 500 mg	500 mg po tid	0.38/500 mg	8	—
Amphotericin B	50 mg vial	50 mg/day IV	11.64/50 mg vial	121	—
Amphotericin B (oral)	100 mg/mL, 24 mL	15 mL qid	27.21/24 mL bottle	27	—
Amphotericin lipid complexes					
Abelcet	100 mg vial	5 mg/kg/d IV	194.00/100 mg	5432	—
AmBisome	100 mg vial	3–5 mg/kg/d IV	188.40/50 mg	9212	—
Amphotec	100 mg vial	3–4 mg/kg/d IV	160.00/100 mg	4480	—
Ampicillin	500 mg cap	500 mg po qid	0.13/500 mg tab	4	8095
Amprenavir (Agenerase)	50, 150 mg caps	1200 mg po bid	1.39/150 mg	156	—
Ativan (Lorazepam)	1 mg tab	1 mg po bid	0.02/1 mg tab	0.28	—
Atovaquone (Mepron)	750 mg/5 mL	750 mg po bid	$11.14/750 mg	222	—
Azithromycin (Zithromax)	250 mg tab	250 mg × 6	6.97/250 mg tab	42	—
	600 mg tab	1200 mg po q wk	16.73/600 mg tab	34	7740
	500 mg vial	500 mg/d	25.23/500 mg vial	175	—

169

Table 38. (continued)

Drug	Formulation	Typical Regimen	AWP[a] Unit Price ($)	Cost/Wk ($)	Cost/Yr ($)[b]
Benadryl (diphenhydramine)	25 mg cap	25 mg HS	0.18/25 mg cap	1	—
Buspar (Buspirone)	5 mg tab	5 mg po tid	0.62/5 mg tab	11	—
Chlorhexidine (Peridex)	480 mL bottle	Oral rinse bid	10.40/480 mL bottle	—	—
Cidofovir (Vistide)	375 mg/5 mL	5 mg/kg IV q2wk	846/375 mg	353	18,356
Ciprofloxacin (Cipro)	250, 500, 750 mg tab	500–750 mg po bid	4.50/750 mg tab	63	—
Clarithromycin (Biaxin)	400 mg vial	400 mg IV bid	28.81/400 mg vial	400	—
	250, 500 mg tab	250–500 mg po bid	3.94/250 mg tab	55	2868
			3.94/500 mg tab	55	
Clindamycin (Cleocin)	300 mg cap	300 mg po qid	1.13/150 mg cap	47	—
	300 mg vial	600 mg IV tid	25.21/600 mg vial	306	—
Clotrimazole (Mycelex)	10 mg troche	10 mg po 5×/d	0.82/10 mg troche	28	1352
Combivir	300 mg AZT + 150 mg 3TC	1 bid	10.33/tab	144	7520
d4T (Stavudine)	15, 20, 30, 40 mg tab	40 mg bid	5.20/40 mg cap	73	3786
Dapsone	100 mg tab	100 mg po qd	0.20/100 mg tab	1	65
ddC (HIVID)	0.375 mg tab 0.75 mg tab	0.75 mg po tid	2.60/0.75 mg tab	55	2883
ddl (Videx)	25, 50, 100, 150 mg tab	200 mg po bid	1.98/100 mg tab	55	2883
ddl (Videx EC)	125, 200, 250, 400 mg	400 mg/d	9.53/400 mg	66	3469
Delavirdine (Rescriptor)	200 mg tab	400 mg po tid	1.63/200 mg tab	68	3560
Doxycycline	100 mg tab	100 mg po bid	0.19/100 mg tab	3	—
Dronabinol (Marinol)	2.5, 5 mg	2.5–5 mg po bid	6.63/5 mg	46–92	4827
Efavirenz (Sustiva)	50, 100, 200 mg caps	600 mg q d	4.39/200 mg cap	93	4836
Erythromycin	250 mg cap	500 mg po qid	0.18/250 mg cap	4	—
Erythropoietin (Procrit, Epogen)	2000, 3000, 4000, 10,000 unit vials	10–30,000 units 3×/wk	$120/10,000 vial	360–1080	—

Drug	How supplied	Dose	Unit cost		
Ethambutol	400 mg tab	400 mg po tid	1.99/400 mg tab	42	2173
Feeding supplements Ensure Sustecal, etc Vivonex TEN	240 mL	240 mL × 4/d	1.50/240 mL	42	1460
Fentanyl patch	1 packet; 25, 50, 75, 100 μg/hr	4 packets/d; 25 μg/hr q 72 h	6.08/packet; 12.20/25 μg/hr	170; 25	8840; —
Fluconazole (Diflucan)	100 mg; 400 mg vial	100 mg po bid; 200 mg IV bid	7.70/100 mg tab; 133.14/400 mg vial	108; 875	5606; —
Flucytosine (5 FC)	250, 500 mg caps	1400 mg/d	2.52/500	247	—
Fluoxetine (Prozac)	10, 20 mg caps	10–40 mg/d	2.83/20 mg cap	20–40	—
Flurazepam (Dalmane)	15, 30 mg caps	15, 30 mg hs	0.06/30 mg cap	1	—
Fomivirsen	330 μg	330 μg q mo	$880/dose	220	2640
Saquinavir soft gel caps (Fortovase)	200 mg caps	6 caps tid	1.09/200 mg cap	133	6945
Foscarnet (Foscavir)	6, 12 g vial; 250 mL vial 5%	6 g IV qd; 60 g IV	73.25/6 g vial; 800/250 mL vial	513; 2100/dose	26,690
Gammaglobulin (Gamimune, etc)					—
Ganciclovir (Cytovene)	500 mg vial	350 mg IV qd	37.10/500 mg vial	170	8800
Ganciclovir oral	250 mg caps	1 g po tid	8.56/500 mg cap	360	18,695
G-CSF (Filgrastim, Neupogen)	300, 480 μg vial	75–300 μg IV or SC qd or qod	300.40/300 μg vial	133–1066	—
Gemfibrozil	600 mg tab	600 mg bid	1.10/600 mg tab	15	800
Growth hormone (Serostim)	6 mg vial	6 mg SC/d	252/6 mg vial	1750	—
Triazolam (Halcion)	0.125, 0.25 mg tab	0.25 mg HS	0.78/0.25 mg tab	5	—
Haloperidol (Haldol)	1 mg tab; 10, 20 μg/mL	2 mg bid	0.55/1 mg tab	2	—
Hepatitis B vaccine		1 mL SC × 3	156/3 doses	—	160
Indinavir (Crixivan)	200, 400 mg	800 mg tid	2.78/400 mg cap	117	6072
Interferon-α (Roferon)	3, 6, 9, 18, 36 mil units vial	3–30 mil units IV or SC qd	11.63/mil units	220–2200	—
Isoniazid (INH)	300 mg tab	300 mg po qd	0.07/300 mg tab	0.50	25
Itraconazole (Sporanox)	100 mg capsule; 100 mg/10 mL oral solution	100 mg po bid; 100 mg/d	7.39/100 mg tab; 7.73/100 mg	103; 54	5380; 2814
Ketoconazole (Nizoral)	100 mg vial; 200 mg tab	100 mg d/IV; 200 mg po qd	100 mg; 3.68/200 mg tab	980; 26–52	1340–2680

Table 38. (continued)

Drug	Formulation	Typical Regimen	AWP[a] Unit Price ($)	Cost/Wk ($)	Cost/Yr ($)[b]
Lamivudine (3TC, Epivir)	150 mg tabs	150 mg bid	4.77/150 mg tab	67	3473
Leucovorin (folinic acid)	5, 10, 15, 25 mg tabs	10 mg po qd	2.85/5 mg tab	40	2080
Levofloxacin (Levaquin)	250, 500 mg tabs	500 mg po qd 500 mg IV qd	17/25 mg tab 8.11/500 mg 39.50/500 mg	119 56 276	6188
Lomotil	2.5 mg tab	5 mg po qid	0.50/2.5 mg tab	18	—
Loperamide (Imodium)	2 mg cap	2 mg 6 × /d	0.65/2 mg	27	—
Lopinavir/ritonavir (Kaletra)	133/33 mg caps	3 caps bid	3.76/cap	284	20,442
Lorazepam	0.5, 1, 2 mg tabs	1–2 mg tid	0.84/2 mg tab	18	—
Megestrol (Megace)	20, 40 mg tab	80 mg qid	1.29/40 mg	72	3588
Methadone	5, 10 mg tab	15–40 mg/d	0.14/10 mg tab	2–3	—
Metronidazole	250, 500 mg tab 500 mg vial	250–500 mg po tid 0.5–1 g IV bid	0.19/250 mg tab 22.39/500 mg vial	4–8 67–134	—
Morphine sulfate (MS contin)	30 mg tab		1.32/30 mg tab		—
Nelfinavir (Viracept)	250 mg tab	750 mg tid/1250 mg bid	2.33/250 mg tab	147–160	7644–8320
Nevirapine (Viramune)	200 mg tab	200 mg po bid	5.04/200 mg tab	71	3669
Nortriptyline (Pamelor)	10, 25, 50 mg tab	75 mg po HS	75 mg caps	2	—
Nystatin	100,000 units/mL	5 u po 5 × /d	0.11/100,000 units	19	1001
Oxandrolone (Oxandrin)	2.5 mg tabs	10–20 mg bid	3.75/2.5 mg	210–420	10,920–21,840
Paromomycin	250 mg caps	500–1 g bid	2.81/250 mg cap	79–158	—
Pentamidine	300 mg vial	300 mg aerosolized q mo	138/300 mg 138/300 mg	25 691	1200
Pneumovax	0.5 mL vial	0.5 mL × 1 SC or IM	13.42/0.5 mL	—	11
Pravastatin	10, 20, 40 mg tabs	20–40 mg/d	2.60/20 mg	18–36	946–1893
Prednisone	50 mg tab	50 mg po qd	0.22/50 mg tab	2	—
Primaquine	15 mg tab	15 mg/d	0.80/15 mg tab	6	—
Prozac (fluoxetine)	10, 20 mg puv	10–40 mg po qd	2.34/20 mg parvule	16–32	—
Pyrazinamide	500 mg tab	500 mg po qid	1.12/500 mg tab	31	1612

Drug	Formulation	Dose	Unit cost	Cost	Annual cost[b]
Pyrimethamine (Daraprim)	25 mg tab	50 mg po qd	0.47/25 mg tab	5	260
Retrovir (AZT, zidovudine)	100, 300 mg	300 mg po bid	5.57/300 mg	78	4055
Rifabutin (Mycobutin)	150 mg cap	300 mg po qd	5.20/150 mg cap	73	3786
Rifampin	300 mg cap	600 mg po qd	2.11/300 mg cap	29	1196
Rifater	50 mg INH, 120 mg Rif, 300 mg PZA	1 tab/10 kg/d	1.80/tab	75	—
Ribavirin (Rebetron)	200 mg cap	5 caps/d	782/84 caps + 6 vials intron	326	—
Methylphenidate (Ritalin)	10 mg tab	10 mg po tid	0.40/10 mg tab	8	—
Ritonavir (Norvir)	100 mg cap	400–600 mg bid	2.06/100 mg cap	116–173	5999–8998
Saquinavir					
Invirase	200 mg cap	400 mg po tid	2.40/200 mg	242	12,580
Fortovase	200 mg cap	400 mg po bid	1.23/200 mg	121	6290
Serostim	4, 5, 6 mg vials	6 mg/d SC	252/mg	1750	—
Sulfadiazine	500 mg tab	0.5–2 g qid	1.02/500 mg tab	28–228	—
Testosterone	100 mg/mL, 10 mL	200–400 mg IM	1.40/100 mg	10	500
Testosterone patch	6 mg	6 mg/d	3.40/patch	24	1238
Trazodone	50, 100, 150, 300 mg tabs	150–300 mg/d	1.41/150 mg tab	10–20	513–1026
Triazolam (Halcion)	0.125, 0.25 mg tab	0.25 mg/d	0.70/0.25 mg tab	5	25
Trimethoprim	100, 200 mg tabs	300 mg tid	0.22/200 mg tab	10	—
Trimethoprim-sulfamethoxazole	DS tab	1 DS po qd	0.14/DS tab	3	51
	16/80 mg/mL vial		1.15/5 mL vial	100	—
Trizivir	AZT + 3TC + ABC	1 bid	16/cap	224	11,648
Valganciclovir (Valcyte)	450 mg tab	900 mg/d	24/tab	336	17,472
Vancomycin	125 mg puvule	125 mg po qid	5.55/125 mg	155	—
	0.5, 1 g vial	1 g bid IV	5.76/500 mg vial	1528	—
Vivonex TEN	1 packet	4 packs po qd	6.20/packet	173	8996

[a] Average wholesale prices (AWP) from PriceAlert, February 15, 2001.

[b] Annual costs are approximate AWP and restricted to drugs given chronically.

Table 39. Adverse Reactions to Antimicrobial Agents Commonly Used in Patients with HIV Infection

	Frequent	Occasional	Rare
Abacavir (Ziagen)		*Hypersensitivity* reaction in 2-3% with fever, GI symptoms ± cough and rash; usually in 1st 6 wk; this is a life-threatening complication in 2-3%; nausea, malaise, diarrhea, anorexia	Lactic acidosis and hepatic steatotosis (class adverse reaction)
Acyclovir (Zovirax)	Initiation at infusion site (IV infusion)	Nausea and vomiting; diarrhea	CNS toxicity with agitation, encephalopathy, disorientation, seizures; hallucinations; anemia; neutropenia; thrombocytopenia; hypotension; rash; renal toxicity especially with prior renal disease; hepatotoxicity; pruritis
Albendazole (Eskazole)		Hepatotoxicity, reversible neutropenia—monitor CBC and liver function tests	
Aminoglycosides Tobramycin Gentamicin Amikacin Netilmicin Kanamycin	Renal failure—dose related: monitor creatinine ≥3×/wk	Vestibular and auditory toxicity—dose related Monitor Romberg and reading after rapid head motion	Fever; rash; blurred vision; neuromuscular blockage; eosinophilia

Drug			
Aminosalicylic acid (PAS)	GI intolerance	Liver damage, allergic reactions, thyroid enlargement	Acidosis, vasculitis, hypoglycemia (diabetes), hypokalemial encephalopathy, decreased prothrombin activity; myalgias, renal damage, gastric hemorrhage
Amprenavir	GI intolerance; rash (15%); oral parenthesias (28%)	Headache, hepatitis Lipodystrophy (class adverse reaction)	Oral prep- 55% propylene glycol—seizures, stupor, disulfiram reactions
Amphotericin B preps (Mayo Clin Proc 73:1205, 1998) *(see comparison table below)*	Fever (maximal at 1 hr) and chills (at 2 hr) (prevent/reduce with hydrocortisone, ibuprofen, ASA, acetaminophen, meperidine); renal damage—dose dependent and reversible in absence of prior renal damage and dose <3 g; reduce with hydration and sodium supplementation; low K+ and Mg++; anemia	Nausea, vomiting, metallic taste, headache, phlebitis at infusion site	Hypotension, rash, pruritus, blurred vision, peripheral neuropathy, convulsions, diabetes insipidus, pulmonary edema, anaphylaxis, acute hepatic failure, eosinophilia, leukopenia, thrombocytopenia
Atovaquone (Mepron)	Rash (20%), nausea (20%), diarrhea (20%); these are sufficiently severe to require discontinuation in 9%	Vomiting, pruritis	Headache, fever, insomnia

Amphotericin B preps (Mayo Clin Proc 73:1205, 1998)

	Ampho B	Ampho colloidal (ABCD)	Ampho B lipid complex (ABCL)	Liposomal ampho B
Infusion toxicity	++++	++	++	–
Renal failure	++++	+	+	+
Hypokalemia	++++	+	+	+
Dose (mg/kg)	1	3–4	5	3–5
Cost/d	30	$500	$700	$1000–1200

Table 39. (continued)

	Frequent	Occasional	Rare
Azithromycin		GI intolerance (dose related) (6%): Diarrhea (4%), reversible ototoxicity (2%), skin rash (1%), headache, fatigue, drowsiness (1%)	Erythema multiforme; increased transaminase Pseudomembranous colitis
Benzodiazepines	Dependency, tolerance, and withdrawal reactions (related to dose and duration): Daytime sedation, dizziness, ataxia	Blurred vision, diplopia, confusion, memory disturbance, amnesia, fatigue, incontinence, constipation, hypotension, bizarre behavior	
Buspirone	CNS: Dizziness, headache, sedation (10%); warn patient	Psychomotor dysfunction, fatigue, anxiety, insomnia (5%); nausea (6–8%); depression (3%); dream disturbance; GI—dry mouth, constipation, diarrhea (1–5%); tachycardia (2%); sexual dysfunction	

Cephalosporins	Phlebitis at infusion sites; diarrhea (especially cefoperazone); pain at IM injection sites (less with cefazolin)	Allergic reactions (anaphylaxis rare): Diarrhea and colitis including C. difficile-associated colitis and PMC; hypoprothrombinemia (cefamandole, cefoperazone, moxalactam, cefmetazole, and cefotetan), eosinophilia, positive Coombs' test	Hemolytic anemia: Interstitial nephritis (cephalothin), hepatic dysfunction, convulsions (high dose with renal failure), neutropenia, thrombocytopenia
Cidofovir	Renal failure—25% develop ≥2 + proteinuria or creatinine increase >2-3 mg/dL (reversible if discontinued). Most give IV hydration and probenecid. Probenecid side effects in 50%: Fever, rash, headache, nausea, GI intolerance—reduce with antiemetics, antipyretics, or antihistamines (Ann Intern Med 1997;126:257)	Neutropenia in 15%, Fanconi syndrome	
Ciprofloxacin (see quinolones)			
Clarithromycin (Biaxin)	GI intolerance (4%), headache (2%), antibiotic-associated diarrhea, transaminase elevation	Rare	

Table 39. (continued)

	Frequent	Occasional	Rare
Clindamycin (Cleocin)	Diarrhea (10–30%)	Nausea, vomiting, anorexia morbilliform, rash, pruritis, C. difficile-associated colitis or PMC	Stevens-Johnson syndrome: Joint pains, neutropenia, thrombocytopenia
Clotrimazole		Oral—increased transaminase (15%), nausea and vomiting (5%). Topical (skin and vaginal)—rash, burning	
Dapsone	Rash, fever, nausea, anorexia, neutropenia—sufficiently severe to require discontinuation in 30–40%; hemolytic anemia (dose dependent)	Blood dyscrasias: methemoglobulinemia and sulfahemoglobinemia ± G-6-PD deficiency, allergic reactions, insomnia, irritability, headache (transient), blurred vision, ringing in ears, hepatitis	Hypoalbuminema; epidermal necrolysis; optic atrophy; aplastic anemia; agranulocytosis; peripheral neuropathy; aplastic anemia; "sulfone syndrome"—fever, exfoliative dermatitis, jaundice, adenopathy, methemoglobinemia, and anemia—treat with steroids; nephrosis
Daunorubicin	Granulocytopenia—monitor CBC predose. Triad of flushing, back pain, and chest tightness—14%; follows infusions and resolves with discontinuation or slowing of infusion	Cardiotoxicity especially with prior cardiac disease or prior treatment with anthracyclines. Monitor ejection fraction with use of large doses (≥320 mg/m²)	Extravasation—tissue necrosis

Delavirdine (Rescriptor)	Rash (18%) maculopapular red, upper body	Headaches Hepatitis	Erythema multiforme, Stevens-Johnson syndrome
Didanosine (ddl: Videx)	GI intolerance 15–20%—diarrhea nausea, vomiting bloating—significantly reduced with Videx EC; *Pancreatitis* (1–9%)—risk is increased with d4T or history of EtoH, prior pancreatitis, low CD4 *Peripheral neuropathy* (5–12%)—rate increased with d4T—reduce dose or discontinue. Note: Na⁺⁺ load of 265 mg/tab and 1350 mg/ powder packet	Hyperuricemia, hepatitis	Lactic acidosis, steatotosis syndrome (class adverse reaction)
Dideoxycytidine (ddC: HIVID)	Peripheral neuropathy 17–31%, frequency is related to cumulative dose, flu-like complaints	Aphthous ulcers, rash, pancreatitis (<1%); hepatitis	Thrombocytopenia, leukopenia, lactic acidosis-hepatic, steatotosis (class adverse reaction)
Doxycycline	GI intolerance (10%), photosensitivity, diarrhea (reduced with food), *Candida* vaginitis		
Dronabinol (Marinol)	Dose related mood high somnolence, confusion (usually resolves with continued use in 1–3 days)	Abuse potential, especially with substance abusers, elderly patients with psychiatric illness, and those receiving sedatives, hypnotics, etc	Hypotension, vasodilation asthenia, tachycardia, visual disturbances

Table 39. (continued)

	Frequent	Occasional	Rare
Efavirenz (Sustiva)	CNS toxicity (53%) with abnormal dreams, confusion, depersonalization, dizziness; usually resolves in 3 wk. Rash (10–15%)— morbilliform, increased serum cholesterol and HDL	Hepatoxicity with elevated transaminase levels	Stevens-Johnson syndrome, lipodystrophy (?)
EPO (epogen, Procrit)		Headache, arthralgias, flu-like illness, GI intolerance, diarrhea fatigue	Hypertension, seizures (?)
Erythromycins	GI Intolerance (oral-dose related); Phlebitis (IV)	Diarrhea, stomatitis, cholestatic hepatitis (especially estolate reversible), generalized rash	Allergic reactions: Colitis, hemolytic anemia, reversible ototoxicity (especially with high doses and renal failure)
Ethambutol (Myambutol)		Optic neuritis: Decreased acuity, reduced color discrimination, constricted fields, scotomata dose related and infrequent with 15 mg/kg/d	Hypersensitivity: Peripheral neuropathy, thrombocytopenia, toxic epidermal neurolysis, lichenoid skin rash

Fentanyl patch	Central nervous system depression and respiratory depression—especially in opiate-naive patients; dose related Tolerance with extended courses Local side effects: Erythema, pruritis, edema at site of application	
Fluconazole (Diflucan)	GI intolerance (2–8%): Rash (5%); transient transaminase (5%) elevation to ≥8 × ULN (1%); headache (2%); diarrhea prolonged protime with coumadin; reversible alopecia × 10–20% with ≥400 mg/d at median of 3 mo after starting (Ann Intern Med 1995;123:354)	Hepatitis, Stevens-Johnson syndrome, thrombocytopenia, anaphylaxis, hypokalemia
Flucytosine	GI intolerance (including nausea, vomiting, diarrhea, and ulcer-active colitis) Marrow suppression with leukopenia or thrombocytopenia (dose related, especially with renal failure, level >100 µg/mL or concurrent amphotericin); confusion; rash: hepatitis (dose related)	Hallucinations, eosinophilia, granulocytosis, fatal hepatitis, peripheral neuropathy
Fluoxetine (Prozac)	GI intolerance (20%), anxiety, agitation insomnia (20%) Headache, tremor, drowsiness, dry mouth, sweating, diarrhea, sexual dysfunction, skin rash	Acute dystonia

Table 39. (continued)

	Frequent	Occasional	Rare
Foscarnet	Dose related renal failure or renal failure reversible)—30% get creatinine >2 mg/dL (monitor creatinine 1–3×/wk and discontinue if creatinine clearance <0.4 mL/min/kg or creatinine >2.9 mg/dL)	Electrolyte changes—reduced Ca^{++}, ionized Ca^{++}, Mg^{++}, PO_4^-, K^+ (8–16%) (monitor electrolytes 1–2×/wk and symptoms—parasthesias and numbness); ionized calcium; seizures (10%); penile ulcers; nausea relieved with slowing infusion or anti-nausea agent	Anemia, thrombocytopenia, wheezing, acute febrile dermatosis (Sweet's syndrome), vasculitis
G-CSF (Neupogen, Filgrastim)	Bone pain in 10–20% (usually controlled with acetaminophen)	Erythema or pain at injection site	
Ganciclovir (Cytovene)	*Neutropenia* with absolute neutrophil count <1000/mm^3 in 25–50% (monitor CBC 2–3×/wk and discontinue if ANC <500/mm^3 or platelet count <25,000/mm^3); dose related	Thrombocytopenia (2–8%); anemia (2%); fever; rash; changes in mental status; abnormal liver function tests (2%); renal failure	Psychosis; neuropathy; impaired reproductive function (?); nausea; vomiting; GI bleeding or perforation; myocardiopathy; encephalopathy
Ganciclovir, oral (Cytovene)	Neutropenia with ANC <500/mm^3 in 18%; anemia with Hgb <8 in 10%; monitor CBC ± treatment with discontinuation or with treatment using G-CSF or GM-CSF	Renal failure (creatinine >2.5 mg/dL in 4%)	

Drug	Adverse Effects	
Haloperidol (Haldol)	CNS: Extrapyramidal symptoms; CNS: Dystonia, motor restlessness; tardive dyskinesia (abrupt withdrawal); sexual dysfunction (10–20%)	Neuroleptic malignant syndrome; hypotension; hepatitis
Hydroxyurea (Hydrea)	Leukopenia and/or anemia—reverses when treatment is discontinued; increases risk of pancreatitis and peripheral neuropathy when used with ddI ± d4T	GI intolerance: Rashes—maculopapular rash, facial erythema, hyperpigmentation; oral ulceration; chronic leg ulcers with use >3 yr; hepatotoxicity	Dysuria, hyperuricemia, renal failure, disorientation chills, fever, alopecia, pancreatitis
Ibuprofen	GI intolerance (give with milk); increased transaminase levels—15%	Peptic ulcer: Bleed or perforation; CNS—dizziness, headache, anxiety; tinnitus	Aseptic meningitis, amblyopia, hearing loss; severe liver toxicity; marrow suppression; renal failure; anaphylaxis
Interferon-α (Roferon, Intron)	Flu-like (80% with 35 mil units/d)—fever, fatigue, anorexia, headache, myalgias; depression—reduce with NSAIDS; GI intolerance (20–65%)—nausea, vomiting, abdominal pain, diarrhea	CNS toxicity: Confusion, paresthias, concentration problems; amnesia; pruritis; marrow supression; alopecia; proteinuria	Delirium, obtundation
Indinavir (Crixivan)	Asymptomatic increase in indirect bilirubinemia (10–15%) Nephrolithiasis 10–20% and nephropathy ascribed to precipitation of drug—must monitor for symptoms and reduce risk with ≥48 oz fluids/d	Dry skin and lips, paronychia; GI intolerance—nausea, vomiting; alopecia may involve any hair site (NEJM 1999;341:618); lipodystrophy (elevated blood lipids, diabetes, and/or fat redistribution)	Metallic taste, fatigue, insomnia, blurred vision, dizziness, rash, thrombocytopenia

Table 39. (continued)

	Frequent	Occasional	Rare
Isoniazid (INH)	Hepatitis—rate increases with age and abuse of alcohol (Ann Intern Med 1999;181: 1014); warn patient; clinical evaluation monthly; D/C if ALT/AST ≥3 × ULN + symptoms or 5× or ≥5× ULN; get baseline LFT and repeat prn	Allergic reactions; fever; peripheral neuropathy—reduce with pyridoxine 50 mg/d; CNS toxicity	CNS—optic neuritis, psychosis, convulsions, nausea, vomiting, myocardiopathy, encephalopathy, blood dyscrasia, lupus-like syndrome, keratitis, pellagra-like rash
Itraconazole (Sporanox)	GI intolerance (5–10%): rash (8%); treatment discontinued in 10%	Pruritis; headaches; asthenia; diarrhea; dizziness; hepatitis (2–3%): impotence (1%)	Fulminant hepatitis (1:1000 and reversible)
Ketoconazole (Nizoral)	GI intolerance (dose related); temporary increase in transaminase levels (2–5%)	Endocrine—decreased steroid and testosterone synthesis with impotence, gynecomastia, oligospermia, reduced libido; menstrual abnormalities (prolonged use and dose related, usually ≥600 mg/d); headache; dizziness; asthenia; pruritis; rash	Abrupt hepatitis (1:15,000): rare cases of fatal hepatic necrosis; anaphylaxis; lethargy; arthralgias; fever; marrow suppression; hypothyroidism (genetically determined); thrombocytopenia; hallucinations
Lamivudine (3TC, Epivir)		Headache, nausea, diarrhea, abdominal pain, insomnia	Lactic acidosis—hepatic steatotosis (class adverse reaction)

Drug		
Levofloxacin (Levaquin)—see quinolones		
Megestrol acetate (Megace)	Sexual dysfunction (estrogen—may respond to testosterone); diarrhea; rash; asthenia; flatulence; pain; GI intolerance; hyperglycemia (5%)	Carpal tunnel syndrome, thrombosis, vaginal bleeding, alopecia, high dose (480–1600 mg/d)—chest pressure, hypertension, dyspnea, congestive heart failure
Lopinavir/ritonavir	Diarrhea in 15–20%; controlled with Imodium or calcium (Tums etc)	Nausea; hepatitis Lipodystrophy with hyperlipidemia, hyperglycemia, and fat redistribution (class adverse reaction)
Metronidazole (Flagyl)	GI intolerance, metallic taste, headache	Peripheral neuropathy (prolonged use, reversible—usually reversible); phlebitis at injection sites; Antabuse-like reaction with alcohol ingestion intolerance (2%) — Seizures; atoxic encephalitis; colitis; leukopenia; dysuria; pancreatitis; allergic reactions; mutagenic in Ames test (clinical relevance as carcinogen with long-term use is unclear); hypotension; ataxia; coma; somnolence
Morphine + other opiate agonists	Tolerance, physical dependence, psychological dependence, withdrawal syndrome (slight with 80 mg MS/d × 30 d; severe with 240 mg MS/d × 30 d)	Acute toxicity: Coma, respiratory depression, cardiac arrest

Table 39. (continued)

	Frequent	Occasional	Rare
Nelfinavir (Viracept)[b]	Diarrhea—10–30%; usually controlled with imodium or calcium (Tums)—sufficiently severe to require discontinuation in 1.6%	Lypodystrophy (elevated blood lipids, diabetes, and/or fat redistribution)	
Nevirapine (Viramune)	Rash (17–30%) usually maculopopular and erythematous ± pruritis; discontinue if rash is severe, accompanied by fever, blisters, or mucous membrane involvement *Hepatotoxicity* in 15–20%; may progress to hepatic necrosis. Most asymptomatic, may have GT 5× or rash. Monitor LFTs esp in first 6 wk	Nausea	Fever, headache Stevens-Johnson syndrome, three rash reactions associated with death (Lancet 1998;351:567)
Nortriptyline and other tricyclics (Pamelor, Aventyl)	Anticholinergic activity; dry mucous membranes, blurred vision, constipation, urinary retention; CNS: Drowsiness, weakness, fatigue	Extrapyramidal symptoms: Tremor, rigidity, dystonia, dysarthria; increased transaminase levels; weight gain; sexual dysfunction; orthostatic hypotension	Neuroleptic malignant syndrome, peripheral neuropathy, ataxia marrow suppression, hepatitis arrhythmias

Nystatin	GI intolerance (nausea, vomiting, diarrhea)
Oxandrolone (Oxandrin)	Virilization in women	Hepatotoxicity, GI intolerance, ankle swelling, insomnia, depression	Peliosis hepatitis (blood filled hepatic cysts)
Paromomycin (Humatin)		GI intolerance, steatorrhea, and malabsorption	Rash, headache, vertigo Aminoglycoside: With GI absorption ± renal failure there could be nephrotoxicity or ototoxicity
Penicillins	Hypersensitivity reactions: Rash (especially ampicillin and amoxicillin); diarrhea (especially ampicillin, amoxicillin, and nafcillin)	GI intolerance (oral agents); fever, Coombs' test positive; phlebitis at infusion sites and sterile abscesses at IM sites; Jarisch-Herxheimer reaction (syphilis or other spirochetal infections)	Anaphylaxis; leukopenia thrombocytopenia; colitis (especially ampicillin) hepatic damage; renal damage; seizures; twitching (high doses in patients with renal failure); hyperkalemia (penicillin G infusion); abnormal platelet aggregation with bleeding diathesis (carbenicillin and ticarcillin)

Table 39. (continued)

	Frequent	Occasional	Rare
Pentamidine (Pentum)	Nephrotoxicity (25%); usually second week of treatment and usually reversible: IM injection: Pain, tenderness, and induration (10–20%)	Hypotension (especially with rapid infusions); hypoglycemia (5–10%), usually after 1 wk, may last days with glucose <25 mg/dL; hyperglycemia and insulin-dependent diabetes; GI intolerance: Nausea, vomiting, abdominal pain, anorexia, and/or bad taste; marrow suppression with leukopenia or thrombocytopenia	Hepatotoxicity, leukopenia, thrombocytopenia, pancreatitis, hypocalcemia, rash, pruritis, fever, urticaria, anaphylaxis, toxic epidermal necrolysis
	Aerosolized administration—cough (in 30%—prevent with Albuterol 2 puffs)	Aerosol administration—asthma reaction (in 5%—prevent with Albuterol, 2 puffs), laryngitis, chest pain	

Drug			
Phenytoin (Dilantin)	Blood levels >25 µg/mL—nystagmus, ataxia, diplopia; >30 µg/mL—lethargy; >50—extreme lethargy	GI intolerance: Gingival hypertrophy; rash; fever; lymphadenopathy. Blood levels >25 µg/mL: Hypotension, vein irritation, inflammation with extravasation, sexual dysfunction; hepatitis. Lab tests: Protime increased, positive LE prep, glucose increased, calcium decreased, thyroid hormones T3 and T4 increased	Dyskinesias, marrow suppression, periarteritis nodosa, acute psychosis
Primaquine		Hemolytic anemia (G-6-PD deficiency)—warn patient to observe for dark urine and/or screen with G-6-PD level pretreatment; GI intolerance—give with meals	Headache, pruritis Methemoglobinemia, hypertension, arrhythmias, disturbed visual accommodation
Pyrazinamide (PZA)	Nongouty polyarthralgia, asymptomatic hyperuricemia	Hepatitis (dose related, frequency not increased when given with INH or rifampin, rarely serious); syndrome of hepatomegaly, fever, and anorexia; GI intolerance; gout (treat with allopurinol or probenecid)	Rash, fever, porphyria, photosensitivity, acute yellow atrophy of liver, acne, skin discoloration, pruritis, sideroblastic anemia, thrombocytopenia

Table 39. (continued)

	Frequent	Occasional	Rare
Pyrimethamine (Daraprim)		Folic acid deficiency with megaloblastic anemia and pancytopenia (dose related and reversed with leucovorin); Allergic reactions (primarily with Fansidar); GI intolerance (reduce dose or give with meals)	CNS—ataxia, tremors, seizures, (dose related), fatigue, headache, depression, insomnia
Quinolones	Animal studies show arthropathies in weightbearing joints of immature animals; significance in humans is unknown, but this class is considered contraindicated in children and during pregnancy	GI intolerance (1–5%); CNS—headache, malaise, insomnia, dizziness; allergic reactions; rash (mild and transient in 1–4%) Candida vaginitis; photosensitivity—sparfloxacin (8%)	Papilledema; nystagmus; visual disturbances; prolonged PT interval; ruptured tendon; PMC; abnormal liver function tests including hepatic necrosis; marrow suppression; photosensitivity; anaphylaxis; seizures; toxic psychosis; CNS stimulation—tremors, restlessness, confusion; arthralgias; interstitial nephritis; renal failure

Rifabutin (Mycobutin)	Note: Uveitis is a dose-related complication seen with >300 mg/d or failure to dose adjust when given with amprenavir, lopinavir, nelfinavir, indinavir, ritonavir or saquinavir, fluconazole. Presentation is a red, painful eye with blurring, photophobia, or floaters. Most respond to topical steroids + mydriatics (NEJM 1994;330:438)	Hepatitis rash (4–10%), leukopenia (3%), thrombocytopenia (usually mild and transient); GI intolerance (5–10%); flu-like illness with interrupted treatment; drug interactions identical to rifampin; dose-related pseudojaundice with yellow skin pigmentation without scleral icterus or elevated bilirubin	Dose-related polyarthralgias; Thrombotic thrombocytopenic purpura; hemolysis; myositis; confusion; seizures
Ribavirin	Hemolytic anemia in first 2 wk		Leukopenia, hyperbilirubinemia, increased uric acid, dyspnea
Rifampin	Orange discoloration of urine, tears (contact lens), sweat	Hepatitis (cholestatic-changes usually in first month of treatment—frequency not increased when given with INH); jaundice (usually reversible with dose reduction and/or continued use); GI intolerance; hypersensitivity reactions (especially with intermittent use); CNS headache, fatigue, confusion, especially in first weeks of treatment; induces cytochrome P-450 to reduce drug levels (see drug interactions); flu-like symptoms with intermittent use characterized by fever, aches ± dyspnea, wheezing	Thrombocytopenia, leukopenia, eosinophilia, hemolytic anemia, renal damage, proximal myopathy, hyperuricemia, anaphylaxis

Table 39. (continued)

	Frequent	Occasional	Rare
Ritonavir (Norvir)	*GI intolerance* (nausea, anorexia, abdominal pain noted in most given standard dose); increased cholesterol and triglycerides Extensive drug interactions	Circumoral and peripheral paresthesias, lypodystrophy—elevated blood lipids, diabetes, fat redistribution (class adverse reaction), hepatitis	
Saquinavir (Fortovase)	*GI intolerance* (nausea, diarrhea, abdominal pain—20–30% of recipients of Fortovase), dose related	Hypoglycemia (3–6%), lypodystrophy elevated blood lipids, diabetes, fat redistribution (class adverse reaction)	Headache, hepatitis, thrombocytopenia, rash
Growth hormone (Serostim)		Fluid and sodium retention with edema, arthralgias, and hypertension; musculoskeletal discomfort (20–50%) with increased tissue turgor and swelling of hands and feet	Flu-like symptoms, rigors, back pain, malaise, carpal tunnel syndrome, chest pain, nausea, diarrhea

Drug			
Stavudine (d4T; Zerit)	Peripheral neuropathy (15–21%), dose related; increased with concurrent ddI	Pancreatitis (0.5–1%), increased pancreatitis when given with ddI or with ddI + hydroxyurea, GI intolerance, headache	Hepatotoxicity, lactic acidosis and hepatic steatotosis (class adverse effect), esophageal ulcers
Sulfonamides	Rash, pruritus, fever, leukopenia	Erythema multiforme, Stevens-Johnson syndrome, serum sickness; crystalluria with renal damage, urolithiasis, and oliguria—dose related and prevented with high output or alkaline urine; GI intolerance; hepatitis	Myocarditis; psychosis; neuropathy; dizziness; depression; hemolytic anemia (G-6-PD deficiency); marrow suppression; ogranulocytosis; photosensitivity
Testosterone (IM)	Androgenic (and anabolic) effects—acne, flushing, virilizing to women, gynecomastia, increased libido, priapsim, edema	Cholestatic hepatitis	
Tetracyclines	GI intolerance (dose related); stains and deforms teeth in children <8 yr; vertigo (minocycline); negative nitrogen balance and increased axotemia with renal failure (except doxycycline); vaginitis	Hepatotoxicity (dose related, especially IV use in pregnant women): esophageal ulcerations; diarrhea; candidiasis (thrush and vaginitis); photosensitivity (especially demeclocycline); phlebitis with IV treatment and pain with IM injection	Malabsorptions; allergic reactions; visual disturbances; aggravation of myasthenia; hemolytic anemia; colitis

Table 39. (continued)

	Frequent	Occasional	Rare
Thalidomide (Thalomid)	100% teratogenic when given at days 35–50 of pregnancy (J Am Acad Dermatol 1996; 35;969) Drowsiness (insomnia was the former indication) Fever and rash in 36%	Dose related paresthesias and extremity pain (may be irreversible); neutropenia	Dizziness, mood changes, bradycardia, bitter taste, pruritus, hypotension
Trazodone (Desyrel)	Sedation in 15–20%	Orthostatic hypotension (5%) Anticholinergic effects—less compared with tricyclics Nervousness, fatigue, dizziness, agitation	Priapism (1/6000)
Trimethoprim	Hyperkalemia in 20–50% given >15 mg/kg/d (NEJM 1993; 328:703). GI intolerance (dose related)	Marrow: Megaloblastic anemia, neutropenia, thrombocytopenia, rash (3%)	Pancytopenia
Trimethoprim-sulfamethoxazole (Bactrim, Septra)	*Fever, leukopenia, pruritis, rash* (AIDS patients: 30–40% required discontinuation, but 60–70% tolerate drug with readministration; dose related)	GI intolerance: Nausea, vomiting, anorexia, diarrheal Candida vaginitis; hepatitis including cholestatic jaundice; anemia; thrombocytopenia; neutropenia; renal failure; erythema multiforme; Stevens-Johnson syndrome; anemia; thrombocytopenia	Ataxis, apathy, ankle clonus, hemolytic anemia owing to G-6-PD deficiency Stevens-Johnson syndrome, erythema multiforme; C. difficile associated colitis or PMC; pancreatitis; hepatic necrosis

Drug			
Vancomycin	Phlebitis at injection site	"Red-man syndrome": Flushing ± dyspnea, urticaria, pruritis, and/or wheezing ascribed to histamine release and directly related to rate of infusion—treat with slowing infusion ± antihistamines, corticosteroids, and/or IV fluids; eosinophilia; allergic reactions with rash; promotes nephrotoxicity and ototoxicity of other drugs especially aminoglycosides	Anaphylaxis; ototoxicity and ? nephrotoxicity (dose related); peripheral neuropathy; marrow suppression
Zidovudine (AZT, Retrovir)	Marrow suppression with anemia or leukopenia related to dose, reversible with discontinuation and/or G-CSF or EPO. Monitor CBC and discontinue with Hgb <8 g/dL or ANC <750/mm³. Macrocytosis not considered a side effect	Subjective complaints with headache, flu-like symptoms, insomnia, and/or myalgias—dose related; myopathy, with extremity weakness and elevated nail pigmentation; GI intolerance—especially nausea	Seizures (reversible): Allergy (rash, anaphylaxis): twitching; mania; hepatitis; cardiomyopathy (ECHO shows decrease EF); lactic acidosis—steatosis (class adverse reaction)

Table 40. Drug Interactions

Drug	Effect of Interaction
Abacavir: None	
Acyclovir	
Narcotics	Increased meperidine levels
Probenecid	Increased acyclovir levels
Albendazole: None	
Amphotericin B	
Aminoglycosides	Increased nephrotoxicity[a]
Capreomycin	Increased nephrotoxicity[a]
Cisplatin	Increased nephrotoxicity
Corticosteroids	Increased hypokalemia
Cyclosporine	Increased nephrotoxicity
Digitalis	Increased cardiotoxicity (monitor K+)
Diuretics	Increased hypokalemia
Methoxyflurane	Increased nephrotoxicity
Skeletal muscle relaxants	Increased effect of relaxants
Vancomycin	Increased nephrotoxicity
Amprenavir (Inhibits cytochrome P450 CYP 3A4 enzymes)	
Abacavir	Increases APV levels 30%—standard doses
Astemizole	Ventricular arrhythmias[a]
Bepridil	Increased bepridil levels[a]
Warfarin (Coumadin)	Increased anticoagulation
Cisapride	Ventricular arrhythmias[a]
Clarithromycin	Increased APV levels 18%—usual doses
Food	High fat meal decreases APV absorption 20%; avoid high fat meal
Ergot alkaloids	Increased ergotamine levels[a]
Ketoconazole	Increase APV levels 31%, ketoconazole levels increased 44%—dose implications unclear
Lovastatin	Increased risk of myopathy[a]
Midazolam	Increased midazolam levels[a]
Rifabutin	Decreases APV AUC 15% and rifabutin AUC increased 200%—use APV standard dose + rifabutin 150 mg qd
Rifampin	Decreases APV AUC 80%[a]
St John's wort	Decreased amprenavir levels[a]
Simvastatin	Increased rates of myopathy[a]
Sildenafil	Increased sildenafil levels—do not exceed 25 mg/48 hr
Terfenadine	Ventricular arrhythmias[a]
Triazolam	Increased triazolam levels[a]
Antiretrovirals	
Efavirenz	EFV increases 15%, APV levels decrease 36%—EFV 600 mg hs + APV 1200 mg tid or APV 1200 mg bid + RTV 200 mg bid + EFV 600 mg hs
Indinavir	IDV levels decrease 38%, APV levels increase 33%—IDV 800 mg tid + APV 800 mg tid
Nelfinavir	NFV levels increase 15%, APV levels increase 1.5×—NFV 750 mg tid + APV 800 mg tid

Table 40. (continued)

Drug	Effect of Interaction
Fortovase	SQV levels decrease 19%, APV levels decrease 32%—Fortovase 800 mg tid + APV 800 mg tid (limited data)
Lopinavir/ritonavir	APV increased, LPV no change—LPV/r 400/100 mg bid + APV 750 mg bid
Atovaquone	
AZT	Increased AZT levels (significance is ?)
Food (fat)	Increased absorption—should be taken with meals
Rifampin and rifabutin	Decreased atovaquone levels[a]
Sulfa-trimethaprim	Decreased TMP-SMX levels (slight)
Tetracycline	Decreased atovaquone levels (40%)
Azithromycin	
Coumadin	Increased prothrombin time
Pimozide	Ventricular arrhythmias[a]
Theophylline	Increased theophylline levels
AZT (Retrovir, Zidovudine)	
Amphotericin B	Increased anemia
Atovaquone	Increased AZT levels
Cancer chemotherapy (adriamycin, vinblastine, vincristine)	Increased marrow toxicity
Clarithromycin	Decreased AZT absorption, give ≥2 hr apart
d4T (Stavudine)	Pharmacologic antagonism
Dapsone	Increased marrow toxicity
Fluconazole (400 mg/d)	Increased AZT levels
Flucytosine	Increased leukopenia
Ganciclovir	Increased leukopenia, concurrent use usually contraindicated except with G-CSF[a]
Interferon	Increased leukopenia
Methadone	Increased AZT levels—no dose adjustment
Phenytoin	Decreased phenytoin levels
Probenecid	Increased AZT levels (and rash)
Rifampin/rifabutin	Decreased AZT levels
Valproate	Possible AZT toxicity
Benzodiazepines	
Caffeine	Antagonizes sedative effect
Cimetidine	Increased benzodiazepine toxicity
Erythromycin	Increased benzodiazepine toxicity
Isoniazid	Increased benzodiazepine toxicity
Omeprazole	Increased benzodiazepine toxicity
Rifampin, rifabutin	Decreased benzodiazepine effect
Cephalosporins	
Alcohol	Disulfiram-like reaction for those with tetrazolethiomethyl side chain: Cefamandole, cefoperazone, cefotetan, cefmetazole
Aminoglycosides	Possibly increased nephrotoxicity
Ethacrynic acid	Increased nephrotoxicity
Furosemide	Increased nephrotoxicity
Probenecid	Increased cephalosporin levels

Table 40. (continued)

Drug	Effect of Interaction
Cidofovir	
Nephrotoxic drugs	Aminoglycosides, amphotericin, foscarnet, IV pentamidine, and non-steroidal antiinflammatory drugs—avoid concurrent use and provide a 7-day ``washout''
Probenecid interactions	Probenecid increases T½ of acyclovir, aminosalicyclic acid, barbiturates, beta-lactams, AZT, benzodiazepines, bumetanide, methotrexate, famotidine, furosemide, theophylline
Clarithromycin	
Carbamazepine (Tegretol)	Increased carbamazepine levels[a]
Cisapride (Propulsid)	Risk of ventricular arrhythmias[a]
Delavirdine	DLV levels increased 44% and clarithromycin levels increased 100%—dose adjust in renal failure
Disopyramide	Increased disopyramide levels[a]
Efavirenz	EFV levels decreased 39% avoid[a]; use azithromycin for MAC
Indinavir	Clarithromycin levels increased 50%—no dose adjustment
Nevirapine	NVP levels increased 26%, clarithromycin levels decreased 30%—standard doses
Pimozide	Risk of ventricular arrhythmia[a]
Rifabutin	Increased rifabutin levels with possible uveitis[a]
Saquinavir	Increased levels of saquinavir
Terfenadine (Seldane)	Risk of ventricular arrhythmias[a]
Theophylline	Elevated theophylline levels
Agents that prolong QT interval	Cisapride, terfenadine, fluoroquinolones—risk of ventricular arrhythmias
Clindamycin	
Antiperistaltic agents (Lomotil, loperamide)	Increased risk and severity of *C. difficile* colitis[a]
Cycloserine	
Alcohol	Increased alcohol effect or convulsions
Ethionamide	Increased CNS toxicity
Isoniazid	CNS toxicity, dizziness, drowsiness
Phenytoin	Increased phenytoin effect (toxicity)
Dapsone	
ddl	Decreased levels of dapsone, give ≥2 hr apart[a]
H₂ blockers, antacids, omeprazole	Decreased absorption of dapsone
Primaquine	Increased hemolysis with G-6-PD deficiency
Probenecid	Increased dapsone levels
Pyrimethamine	Increased marrow toxicity (monitor CBC)
Rifampin and rifabutin	Decreased levels of dapsone
Saquinavir	Increased dapsone levels
Trimethoprim	Increased levels of both drugs
Warfarin (Coumadin)	Increased prothrombin time

Table 40. (continued)

Drug	Effect of Interaction
d4T (Stavudine)	
AZT	Pharmacologic antagonism
ddC and ddl	Increased peripheral neuropathy and possible increase in acute pancreatitis especially when d4T is combined with ddl and hydroxyurea
Agents associated with peripheral neuropathy	Increased frequency and severity of peripheral neuropathy: Cisplatin, dapsone, ddl, ddC, disulfiram, ethionamide, glutethimide, gold, hydralazine, iodoquinol, INH, phenytoin, metronidazole (long term), vincristine
ddC (HIVID, zalcitabine, dideoxycytidine)	
ddl and d4T	Increased peripheral neuropathy[a]
Agents associated with peripheral neuropathy	Increased frequency and severity of peripheral neuropathy: Cisplatin, dapsone, ddl, ddC, d4T, disulfiram, ethioinamide, glutethimide, gold, hydralazine, INH, iodoquinol, metronidazole, nitrofurantoin, phenytoin, vincristine[a]
Agents associated with pancreatitis	Pentamidine, ddl, rifampin, alcohol abuse
ddl (Videx, didanosine)	
Note: All drugs that require gastric acidity for absorption should be given ≥2 hr before or after buffered ddl. This does *not* apply to Videx EC (enteric coated ddl). The following applies only to buffered ddl	
Dapsone	Decreased dapsone absorption, give ≥2 hr before ddl[a]
Delavirdine	Decreased delavirdine absorption, give ≥2 hr apart
Ganciclovir—oral	Increased ddl levels 70% (may require ddl dose reduction)
Ketoconazole, itraconazole	Decreased ketoconazole or itraconazole absorption, give ≥2 hr before ddl[a]
Indinavir	Decreased indinavir absorption, give ≥2 hr apart
Quinolones	Decreased quinolone absorption, give ≥2 hr before ddl[a]
Ritonavir	Decreased ritonavir absorption, give ≥2 hr apart
Tetracycline	Decreased tetracycline absorption, give ≥2 hr before ddl[a]
ddl buffered and enteric coated (Videx EC)	
Drugs that cause peripheral neuropathy (use with caution)	Ethambutol, INH, vincristine, gold, disulfiram, cisplatin, d4T, hydroxyurea
Ganciclovir	ddl levels increased 100%; monitor for ddl toxicity
Methadone	ddl levels decreased 41%—dose implications unclear

Table 40. (continued)

Drug	Effect of Interaction
d4T	
Agents associated with pancreatitis	Pentamidine, rifampin, alcohol abuse, ddI, hydroxyurea
Agents associated with peripheral neuropathy	Increased frequency and severity of peripheral neuropathy: Cisplatin, dapsone, ddC, d4T, disulfiram, ethioinamide, glutethimide, gold, hydralazine, iodoquinol, INH, metronidazole, nitrofurantoin, phenytoin, vincristine
Dronabinol (Marinol)	
Alcohol	Increased CNS depression
Amitriptyline, amoxapine, other tricyclic antidepressants	Tachycardia, hypertension, drowsiness
Amphetamines, cocaine, and other sympathomimetic drugs	Increased hypertension and tachycardia
Atropine, scopolamine, and other anticholingergic agents	Tachycardia, drowsiness
Efavirenz (induces and inhibits CYP3A)	
Astemizole	Ventricular arrhythmias[a]
Carbamazepine	Decreased levels of EFV
Cisapride	Ventricular arrhythmias[a]
Clarithromycin	Decrease clarithromycin levels 39%[a]; rash in 46%—avoid[a]
Ergot alkaloids	Increased ergot levels[a]
Ethinyl estradiol	Increased levels estradiol by 37%—use alternative method
Methadone	Methadone levels reduced monitor for withdrawal
Midazolam	Increased levels midazolam[a]
Phenobarbital	Decreased levels EFV
Phenytoin	Decreased levels EFV
Rifabutin	Rifabutin levels decreased 35% and EFV levels are unchanged; use rifabutin 450 mg–600 mg/d or 100 mg 2 ×/wk + EFV 600 mg/d
Rifampin	EFV levels decreased 25%—no dose change
Terfenadine	Risk of arrhythmias[a]
Triazolam	Increased triazolam levels[a]
Antiretrovirals	
Amprenavir	APV levels decreased 36%, EFV no change—APV 1200 mg tid + EFV 600 mg/d or APV 1200 mg 1200 bid + RTV 200 mg bid + EFV 600 mg/d
Indinavir	IDV levels decreased 31%, EFV shows no change—IDV 1000 mg tid + EFV 600 mg/d
Lopinavir/ritonavir	LPV levels decreased 29%, EFV no change—EFV 600 mg hs + LPV/r 533/133 (4 caps) bid
Nelfinavir	NFV increased 20%, EFV unchanged—NFV 750 mg tid or 1250 mg bid + EFV 600 mg/d
Ritonavir	RTV increased 18%, EFV increased 21%—RTV 500–600 mg bid + EFV 600 mg/d

Table 40. (continued)

Drug	Effect of Interaction
Saquinavir	SQV decreased 62% and EFV decreased 12%—contraindicated

Erythromycins (inhibit cytochrome P450 enzymes)

Anticoagulants (oral)	Increased hypoprothrombinemia
Carbamazepine	Increased carbamazepine levels
Corticosteroids	Increased effect of methylprednisolone
Cyclosporine	Increased cyclosporine levels (nephrotoxicity)
Digoxin	Increased digitalis levels
Disopyramide	Increased disopyramide toxicity[a]
Ergot alkaloids	Increased ergot toxicity[a]
Felodipine	Increased felodipine levels
Phenytoin	Increased phenytoin levels
Propulsid (cisapride)	Ventricular arrhythmias[a]
Tacrolimus	Increased tacrolimus levels
Terfenadine (Seldane)	Ventricular arrhythmias[a]
Theophylline	Increased theophylline levels
Triazolam	Increased triazolam levels
Valproate	Increased valproate levels
Agents that prolong QT interval—cisapride, terfenadine, quinidine, amioderone, fluoroquinolones	Ventricular arrhythmias

Erythropoietin (EPO)   None

Ethambutol

Al-containing drugs	May decrease absorption

Famciclovir

Cimetidine	Increased penciclovir levels
Digoxin	Increased digoxin levels
Probenecid	Increased penciclovir levels
Theopylline	Increased penciclovir levels

Fluconazole (inhibits cytochrome P-450)

Alprazolam	increased sedation
Atovaquone	Increased atovaquone levels
AZT	Increased AZT levels with fluconazole doses ≥400 mg/d
Benzodiazepines	Increased benzodiazepine levels
Cisapride	Ventricular arrhythmias
Clarithromycin	Increased clarithromycin levels
Contraceptives	Decreased contraception effect—three cases reported
Cyclosporine	Increased cyclosporine levels
Midazolam	Increased sedation
Nortriptyline	Increased sedation and ventricular arrythmias

Table 40. (continued)

Drug	Effect of Interaction
Opiate analgesics	Increased opiate effect
Phenytoin	Increased phenytoin levels
Propulsid (cisapride)	Ventricular arrhythmias[a]
Rifabutin	Increased rifabutin levels with possible uveitis[a]
Saquinavir	Increased saquinavir levels (advantage)
Sulfonylureas	Increased levels with hypoglycemia
Terfenadine (Seldane)	Ventricular arrhythmias[a]
Warfarin (Coumadin)	Increased prothrombin time

Fluoroquinolones (ciprofloxacin, norfloxacin, ofloxacin, lomefloxacin, enoxacin, levofloxacin, moxifloxacin, gatifloxacin)

Drug	Effect of Interaction
Antacids	Decreased fluoroquinolone absorption with Mg-, Ca-, or Al-containing antacids or sucralfate: Give antacid >2 hr after fluoroquinolone
Anticogulants (oral)	Increased hypoprothrombinemia
Caffeine	Increased caffeine effect; primarily with ciprofloxacin and enoxacin; significance?
Cyclosporine	Possible increased nephrotoxicity
Food (dairy product)	Decreased absorption
Iron	Decreased ciprofloxacin absorption[a]
Nonsteroidal anti-inflammatory agents	Possible seizures and increased epileptogenic potential of theophylline, opiates, tricyclics, and neuroleptics
Probenecid	Increased fluoroquinolone levels
Theophylline	Increased theophylline toxicity, especially ciprofloxacin and enoxacin (seizures, cardiac arrest, respiratory failure caused by theophylline toxicity)[a]
Zinc	Decreased ciprofloxacin absorption
Agents that prolong QT interval—erythromycin, clarithromycin, amioderone, quinidine, procainamide, cisapride	Ventricular arrhythmias

Fluoxetine (Prozac)

Drug	Effect of Interaction
Astemizole	Increased astemizole levels
Digitalis	Increased digitalis levels
Haloperidol	Increased haloperidol levels
MAO inhibitors	Risk of serotonergic syndrome—avoid initiating fluoxetine until ≥14 days after discontinuing MAO inhibitor
Saquinavir	Increased saquinavir levels
Terfenadine (Seldane)	Ventricular arrhythmias[a]
Theophylline	Increased theophylline levels
Tricyclics	Increased tricyclic levels
Warfarin (Coumadin)	Increase prothrombin time

Table 40. (continued)

Drug	Effect of Interaction
Foscarnet	
Aminoglycosides	Increased renal toxicity
Amphotericin B	Increased renal toxicity
Imipenem	Increased frequency of seizures (?)
Pentamidine	Increased hypocalcemia and renal toxicity[a]
Ganciclovir	
AZT (Retrovir)	Increased leukopenia, concurrent use should be used with caution, may need G-CSF
Imipenem	Increased frequency of seizures (?)
Myelosuppressing drugs: TMP-SMX, AZT, azathrioprine, pyrimethamine, flucytosine, interferon, adriamycin, vinblastine, vincristine	Increased neutropenia
Probenecid	Increased ganciclovir levels
Ganciclovir, oral	
AZT	Increased neutropenia
ddl	Decreased absorption take ≥2 hr apart
Food	Increased ganciclovir levels—should be taken with meals
Myelosuppressing drugs	See above
G-CSF and GM-CSF	
Cancer chemotherapy	Should not be given within 24 hr of chemotherapy
Indinavir (inhibits P-450 3A4 enzymes)	
Anticonvulsants	Decreased indinavir levels
Astemizole	Increased astemizole levels, cardiac arrhythmias[a]
Cisapride	Increased cisapride levels[a]
Clarithromycin	Clarithromycin in levels increased 50%—no dose adjustment
Didanosine (ddl)	Decreased indinavir absorption, take ≥2 hr apart
Ergot alkaloids	Increased ergot levels[a]
Estradiol	Estradiol levels increased 24%—no dose adjustment
Food	Decreased indinavir levels—take on empty stomach or with light meal without fat
Grapefruit juice	Decreased indinavir levels 26%
Ketoconazole	Increased levels of indinavir; reduce indinavir dose to 600 mg q8h
Lovastatin	Increased lovastatin levels[a]
Methadone	No change in levels
Midazolam (Versed)	Increased midazolam levels[a]

Table 40. (continued)

Drug	Effect of Interaction
Rifampin and rifabutin	Decreased indinavir levels and increased levels of rifampin or rifabutin, avoid rifampin; reduce rifabutin to half dose and increase indinivar dose to 1000 mg tid
St John's wort	Decreased IDV levels[a]
Simvastatin	Increased simvastatin levels[a]
Sildenafil	Increased levels of sildenafil—do not exceed 25 mg/48 hr
Terfenadine (Seldone)	Increased terfenadine levels with cardiac arrhythmias[a]
Triazolam (Halcion)	Increased triazolam levels[a]
Antiretrovirals	
Delavirdine	Increase IDV levels 2 × —IDV 600 mg q8h + DLV 400 mg bid
Efavirenz	IDV decreased 31% EFV no effect—IDV 1000 mg q 8 h + EFV 600 mg/d
Amprenavir	APV increased 31%, IDV decreased 38%—APV 800 mg tid + IDV 800 mg tid
Lopinavir/ritonavir	LPV—no change, IDV increased 3× —IDV 600 mg bid + LPV/r 400/100 mg bid
Nelfinavir	NFV levels increased 80%, IDV increased 50%—IDV 1200 mg bid + NFV 1250 mg bid
Nevirapine	IDV levels decreased 10–30%—IDV 1000 mg tid + NVP standard
Ritonavir	Increases in levels of both drugs—IDV 400 mg bid + RTV 400 mg bid or IDV 800 mg bid + RTV 100–200 mg bid
Saquinavir (Invirase)	Increased SQV levels 4–7 × (advantage)
Interferon	
AZT	Increased marrow suppression
Barbiturates	Increased barbiturate levels
Theophylline	Increased theophylline levels
Isoniazid	
Alcohol	Increased hepatitis
	Decreased INH effect in some alcholics
Antacids	Decreased INH levels with Al-containing antacids
Benzodiazepines	Increased effects of benzodiazepines
Carbamazepine	Increased toxicity of both drugs[a]
Cycloserine	Increased CNS toxicity, dizziness, drowsiness
Diazepam	Increased diazepam levels—reduce diazepam dose
Disulfiram	Psychotic episodes, ataxia[a]
Ethionamide	Increased CNS toxicity
Enflurane	Possible nephrotoxocity[a]
Food	Decreased absorption
Ketoconazole or itraconazole	Decreased azole effect[a]
Phenytoin	Increased phenytoin toxicity
Rifampin and rifabutin	Possible increased hepatic toxicity
Theophylline	Increased theophylline levels

Table 40. (continued)

Drug	Effect of Interaction
Tyramine (foods and fluids rich in tyramine—especially cheese, wine, some fish)	Rare patients get palpitations, sweating, urticaria, headache, and/or vomiting
Warfarin (Coumadin)	Increased hypoprothrombinemia
Itraconazole (inhibits cytochrome P-450)	Note: caps require gastric acid and should be taken with food; liquid suspension should be taken on empty stomach and does not require acid
Alprazolam	Increased sedation
Astemizole	Increased astemizole levels[a]
Calcium channel blockers	Increased levels of Ca blocker
Carbamazepine (Tegretol)	Decreased itraconazole levels
Cisapride	Ventricular arrhythmias[a]
Coke and other acidic drinks	Increased absorption of caps
Contraceptives	Decreased contraceptive effect
Cyclosporine	Increased cyclosporine levels
ddl	Decreased itraconazole levels—take ≥2 hr apart or use Videx EC
Digoxin	Increased digoxin levels
Food	Increased itraconazole absorption; give with meal
H₂ antagonists, antacids, omeprazole, sucralfate	Decreased itraconazole levels—does not apply to oral itraconazole solution
Hypoglycemics, oral	Severe hypoglycemia
Indinavir	Increased IDV levels—decrease IDV dose to 600 mg tid
Isoniazid	Decreased itraconazole levels[a]
Lovastatin	Increased myopathy risk[a]
Midazolam	Increased midazolam levels[a]
Phenobarbitol	Decreased itraconazole levels[a]
Phenytoin	Decreased itraconazole levels[a]
Cisapride (Propulsid)	Ventricular arrhythmias[a]
Rifampin or rifabutin	Decreased itraconazole levels[a]
Simvastatin	Increased myopathy risk[a]
Terfenadine (Seldane)	Ventricular arrhythmias[a]
Triazolam	Increased triazolam effect[a]
Warfarin (Coumadin)	Increased hypoprothrombinemia
Ketoconazole (inhibits cytochrome P-450)	
Alcohol	Possible disulfiram-like reaction
Alprazolam	Increased sedation
Amprenavir	APV levels increased 31% and ketoconazole levels decreased 44%—dose implications unclear
Antacids	Decreased ketoconazole levels
Astemizole	Ventricular arrhythmia[a]
Cisapride	Increased cisapride levels, ventricular arrhythmias[a]
Contraceptives	Decreased contraceptive effect
Corticosteroids	Increased methylprednisolone levels
Cyclosporine	Increased cyclosporine toxicity
ddl	Decreased ketoconazole levels—give ≥2 hr apart
Efavirenz	Not studied
Food	Decreased ketoconazole absorption—give ≥2 hr apart

Table 40. (continued)

Drug	Effect of Interaction
H$_2$ antagonists, antacids, omeprazole	Decreased ketoconazole levels[a] (use sucralfate or take antacids more than 2 hr before)
Hypoglycemics, oral	Severe hypoglycemia
Indinavir	Increased indinavir levels 70%; reduce indinavir dose to 600 mg q8h
Isoniazid	Decreased ketoconazole levels[a]
Lopinavir	Ketoconazole levels increased 3×—dose implications unclear
Loratadine (Claritin)	Increased levels of loratadine
Midazolam	Increased midazolam levels[a]
Nelfinavir	No dose change
Nevirapine	NVP levels increased 15–30%, ketoconazole levels decreased 63%—avoid[a]
Phenytoin	Altered metabolism of both drugs
Rifampin and rifabutin	Decreased activity of both drugs[a]
Ritonavir	Increase ketoconazole levels 3×; do not exceed 200 mg/d
Saquinavir	Increased saquinavir levels by 150% (advantage)
Terfenadine (Seldane)	Ventricular arrhythmias[a]
Theophylline	Increased theophylline levels
Triazolam	Increased triazolam levels[a]
Warfarin (Coumadin)	Increased hypoprothrombinemia
Lamivudine (3TC, Epivir)	
AZT	Resistance to 3TC promotes susceptibility to AZT—advocated combination
Trimethoprim	Increases 3TC levels 40% (implications unclear)
Megestrol	None
Methadone	
AZT	Increased AZT levels 44%—no dose adjustment
Alcohol	Increased CNS depression
ddI	Reduces ddI levels 60%[a]
Dronabinol (Marinol)	Increased CNS depression
Efavirenz	Reduction in methadone levels with opiate withdrawal—use with caution or increase methadone dose
Indinavir	No changes
Lopinavir	Decreased methadone AUC 53%; monitor for withdrawal
Marijuana	Increased CNS depression
Nelfinavir	Methadone levels decreased; monitor for withdrawal
Nevirapine	Reduces methadone levels 60%—avoid or increase methadone dose
Rifampin and rifabutin	Reduced methadone levels
Ritonavir	Reduced methadone levels 36%—consider increase in methadone dose
Saquinavir	No data

Table 40. (continued)

Drug	Effect of Interaction
Metronidazole	
Alcohol	Disulfiram-like reaction
Barbiturates	Decreased metronidazole effect with phenobarbital
Cimetidine	Possible increased metronidazole levels
Corticosteroids	Decreased metronidazole levels
Disulfiram	Organic brain syndrome[a]; stop disulfiram 2 wk before metronidazole
Flurouracil	Transient neutropenia
Food	Reduces gastric irritation
Lithium	Lithium toxicity
Cisapride (Propulsid)	Ventricular arrhythmias[a]
Terfenadine (Seldane)	Ventricular arrhythmias[a]
Coumadin (Warfarin)	Increased hypoprothrombinemia
Lopinavir/ritonavir	Inhibits P450 isoenzymes
Astemizole	Risk of arrhythmias[a]
Atorvastatin	Atorvastatin AUC increased $6\times$[a]
Cisapride	Risk of arrhythmias[a]
Ergot derivatives	Increased ergot levels[a]
Ethyl estradiol	Ethyl estradiol AUC decreased 42%—use alternative method
Ketoconazole	Ketoconazole levels increased $3\times$—implications unclear
Methadone	Methadone AUC decreased 53%; monitor for withdrawal
Midazolam	Risk of arrhythmias[a]
Pimozide	Risk of arrhythmias
Rifabutin	Rifabutin levels increased $5\times$—decrease RBT dose to 150 mg qod + standard LPV/r dose
Rifampin	Lopinavir levels decreased[a]
Terfenadine	Risk of arrhythmias[a]
Triazolam	Risk of arrhythmias[a]
Nelfinavir (Viracept) (inhibits CYP 3A4 enzymes)	
Astemizole	Ventricular arrhythmias[a]
Cisapride	Ventricular arrhythmias[a]
Ergot alkaloids	Increased ergot levels[a]
Ethinyl estradiol	Decreased levels; use alternative method of birth control
Lovastatin	Risk of myopathy[a]
Methadone	Methadone levels decreased but standard doses
Midazolam	Increased midazolam levels[a]
Rifabutin	NFV levels decreased 32%, RBT levels increased $2\times$—NFV 1000 mg tid RBT 150 mg q d reduction by 50% (150 mg QD); nelfinavir levels reduced 32%—increase NFV dose to 1000 mg tid
Rifampin	Reduces nelfinavir levels 82%—avoid[a]

Table 40. (continued)

Drug	Effect of Interaction
Simvastatin	Risk of myopathy[a]
St John's wort	Decreased NFV levels[a]
Sildenafil	Increased sildenafil levels—do not exceed 25 mg/48 hr
Terfenadine	Ventricular arrhythmias[a]
Triazolam	Increased levels of triazolam[a]
Antiretroviral drugs	
Amprenavir	NFV levels increased 15%, APV increased 1.5× —NFV 750 mg bid + APV 800 mg tid (limited data)
Delavirdine	Levels 2× and decreased delavirdine levels 50%—NFV 1250 mg bid, DLV 600 mg bid for neutropenia
Efavirenz	No data
Indinavir	Nelfinavir levels increased 80%, IDV levels increased 50%—IDV 1000 mg bid + NFV 1250 mg bid
Lopinavir/ritonavir	No data
Nevirapine	NFV increase 10%, NVP no effect—standard doses
Ritonavir	Nelfinavir levels increased 1.5×, RTV levels unchanged—RTV 400 mg bid + NFV 500–750 mg bid
Saquinavir	Nelfinavir levels increased 20%; saquinavir levels increased 3× —NFV standard + Fortovase 800 mg tid or 1200 mg bid
Nevirapine	Induces cytochrome P-450 enzymes
Methadone	Reduces methadone levels—monitor methadone dose
Antirotroviral drugs	
Amprenavir	No data
Indinavir	IDV decreased 28%, NVP unchanged, IDV 1000 mg q8h + NVP standard
Lopinavir/ritonavir	LPV decreased 50%, NVP no change—LPV/r 533/133 mg bid + NVP standard dose
Nelfinavir	NFV levels increased 10%, NFV unchanged—standard dose
Ritonavir	RTV decreased 11%, NVP no effect—standard dose
Saquinavir	SQV levels decreased 25%, NVP no effect—not recommended
Nortriptyline	
Adrenergic blockers	Increase adrenergic block
Cimetidine	Increased nortriptyline levels
Clonidine	Increased clonidine level
Fenfluramine	Increased fenfluramine levels
Fluconazole	Increased nortriptyline levels
MAO inhibitors	Increased levels of MAO inhibitors[a]
Quinidine	Increased nortriptyline levels

Table 40. (continued)

Drug	Effect of Interaction
Nystatin	None
Oxandrolone	
Hypoglycemics, oral	Increased hypoglycemia
Warfarin (Coumadin)	Increased anticoagulation
Paromomycin	None
Penicillins	
Allopurinol	Increased frequency of rash with ampicillin
Contraceptives	Possible decreased contraceptive effect with ampicillin or oxacillin
Cyclosporine	Decreased cyclosporine effect with nafcillin and increased cyclosporine toxicity with ticarcillin
Food	Decreased absorption (oral penicillin G)[a]
Lithium	Hypernatremia with ticarcillin
Methotrexate	Possible increased methotrexate toxicity
Probenecid	Increased concentrations of penicillins
Warfarin	Decreased anticoagulant effect with nafcillin and dicloxacillin
Pentamidine (IV)	
Aminoglycosides	Increased nephrotoxicity[a]
Amphotericin B	Increased nephrotoxicity[a]
Capreomycin	Increased nephrotoxicity[a]
ddI	Increased risk of pancreatitis
Foscarnet	Increased nephrotoxicity[a]
Pyrazinamide	None
Pyrimethamine	
Antacids	Possible decreased pyrimethamine absorption
Dapsone	Agranulocytosis reported
Ganciclovir	Increased neutropenia
Kaolin	Possible decreased pyrimethamine absorption
Lorazepam	Hepatotoxicity
Phenothiazines	Possible chlorpromazine toxicity

Rifabutin (induces cytochrome P-450 for increased hepatic metabolism; effect is less pronounced compared with rifampin; both drugs are also metabolized by cytochrome P-450 3A4 so drugs that inhibit these enzymes prolong the half-life of rifabutin and rifampin); see below for drug interaction affected by this mechanism

Table 40. (continued)

Drug	Effect of Interaction
See listing for rifampin	
Clarithromycin	Increased rifabutin levels and risk of uveitis[a]
Fluconazole	Increased rifabutin levels and risk of uveitis[a]
Antiretroviral agents	
Ritonavir	Increased rifabutin levels and decreased ritonavir levels—RBT 150 mg qod + RTV standard
Indinavir	Increased rifabutin levels—RBT 150 mg/d + IDV 1000 mg q8h rifabutin dose 50% (150 mg/d) and increase IDV to 1200 mg tid
Saquinavir	Increased rifabutin levels, reduced saquinavir levels; concurrent use is contraindicated[a]
Nelfinavir	Increased rifabutin levels and reduced NFV—RBT 150 mg/d + NFV 1000 mg tid
Amprenavir	Rifabutin levels increased and AMP level decreased—RBT 150 mg/d + APV standard
Efavirenz	Rifabutin levels decreased 32% and EFV levels are unchanged—RBT 450–600 mg/d + EFV standard dose
Delavirdine	Decrease DLV levels 80%—contraindicated[a]
Nevirapine	Decreased levels both drugs—NVP 200 mg bid + RBT 300 mg qd
Ritonavir + saquinavir	SQV levels decrease, RBT levels increase 3×—RTV 150 mg 2–3×/wk
Lopinavir + ritonavir	RBT levels increase 5×, LPV unchanged—LPV/r standard, RBT 150 qod
Rifampin (induces cytochrome P-450 hepatic enzymes; also metabolized by cytochrome P-450 enzymes)	
Aminosalicyclic acid (PAS)	Decreased effectiveness of rifampin; give in separate doses × 8–12 hr
Antiretroviral agents	Levels of delavirdine, amprenavir, indinavir, nelfinavir, lopinavir, and saquinavir are decreased; concurrent use is contraindicated with the following exceptions: Ritonavir and saquinavir, efavirenz, and possibly nevirapine
Atovaquone	Decreased atovaquone levels
Barbiturates	Decreased barbiturate levels
Benzodiazepines	Possible decreased benzodiazepine levels
Beta-adrenergic blockers	Decreased beta-blocker levels
Chloramphenicol	Decreased chloramphenicol levels[a]
Clofibrate	Decreased clofibrate levels
Contraceptives	Decreased contraceptive effect[a]
Corticosteroids	Decreased corticosteroid levels[a]

Table 40. (continued)

Drug	Effect of Interaction
Ciprofloxacin	Increased RBT levels
Clarithromycin	Increased RBT levels
Cyclosporine	Decreased cyclosporine levels[a]
Dapsone	Decreased dapsone levels
Digitalis	Decreased digitalis levels
Disopyramide	Decreased disopyramide levels[a]
Doxycycline	Decreased doxycycline levels
Erythromycin	Increased RBT levels
Estrogens	Decreased estrogen effect; use alternative method of birth control
Fluconazole	Decreased fluconazole levels; increased RBT levels
Food	Decreased rifampin absorption
Haloperidol	Decreased haloperidol levels
Hypoglycemics	Decreased hypoglycemic effect
Isoniazid	Increased hepatoxicity
Itraconazole	Increased RBT levels
Ketoconazole	Decreased levels of both drugs[a]; increased RBT levels
Methadone	Methadone withdrawal symptoms[a]
Mexiletine	Decreased antiarrhythnmic effect
Nifedipine	Decreased antihypertensive effect
Phenytoin	Decreased phenytoin levels
Progestins	Decreased norethindron levels
Quinidine	Decreased quinidine levels
Theophylline	Decreased theophylline levels
Trimethoprim	Decreased trimethoprim levels
Triazolam	Decreased triazolam levels
Trimetrexate	Decreased trimetrexate levels
Verapamil	Decreased verapamil levels
Warfarin (coumadin)	Decreased hypoprothrombinemia

Ritonavir (profound inhibition of P-450 cytochromes including 3A and 2D6; this is also the major mechanism of ritonavir metabolism). Drugs that should *not* be co-administered: Encainide amiodarone, flecainide, propafenone, quinidine, bepridil (Vascor), astemizole, simvastatin, lovastatin, terfenadine (Seldane), cisapride (Propulsid), midazolam (Versed), triazolam (Halcion), pimozide, St John's wort, and ergot alkaloids

Carbamazepine	Decreased ritonavir levels
Clarithromycin	Increase clarithromycin levels 77%—reduce dose in renal failure
Desipramine	Increased desipramine levels—monitor levels of desipramine
Didanosine (ddl)	Reduced ritonavir absorption; take ≥2 hr apart
Ethinyl estradiol	Ethinyl estradiol levels decreased 40%—use alternative method
Erythromycin	Increased erythromycin levels
Fentanyl	Increased fentanyl levels
Food	Modest increase in ritonavir levels—take with meals
Ketoconazole	Increased ketoconazole levels—do not exceed 200 mg/d

Table 40. (continued)

Drug	Effect of Interaction
Methadone	Methadone levels decreased 39%, consider dose increase
PIs and NNRTIs	
Amprenavir	APV levels increase 2.5× —APV 600–1200 mg bid + RTV 100–200 mg bid or APV 1200 mg/d + RTV 200 mg qd
Delavirdine	No data
Efavirenz	Levels RTV increase 18%, EFV levels increase 21%—RTV 600 mg bid + EFV 600 mg/d
Indinavir	IDV levels increase 2–5× —IDV 400 mg bid, RTV 400 mg bid
Lopinavir/efavirenz	LPV levels decrease 40%, EFV unchanged—LLV/r 533/133 mg bid + EFV 600 mg/d
Nelfinavir	NFV increase 1.5 × —NFV 500–750 mg bid + RTV 400 mg bid
Nevirapine	No significant interaction—standard doses of each
Saqunavir	SQV levels increase 20× —RTV 400 mg bid + SQV 400 mg bid or RTV 100 mg qd + SQV 1600 mg qd
Oral contraceptives	Reduced estradiol levels 40%; use alternative method of contraception
Oxycodone	Increased oxycodone levels
Phenobarbitol	Decreased ritonavir levels
Phenytoin	Decreased ritonavir levels
Rifabutin	Rifabutin levels increase 4×, decrease rifabutin dose to 150 mg qod + RTV standard dose
Rifampin	RTV levels decrease 35%, use standard doses both drugs
Sildenafil	Increased levels of sildenafil with potential for increased side effects—do not exceed 25 mg/48 hr
St John's wort	Decreased levels RTV[a]
Theophylline	Reduced theophylline levels 43%—monitor theophylline levels
Tricyclic antidepressants	Moderate increased tricyclic levels
Warfarin	Increased anticoagulant effect
Saquinavir	Inhibition of CYP 34A enzyme
Astemizole	Increase levels of both drugs[a]
Carbamazepine	Decreased saquinavir levels
Cisapride	Increased cisapride levels[a]
Clarithromycin	Increased clarithromycin 45%, SQV levels increased 177%—with SQV + RTV use clarithromycin 150 mg 2–3×/wk
Clindamycin	Increased clindamycin levels
Dapsone	Increased dapsone levels
Dexamethasone	Decrease saquinavir levels

Table 40. (continued)

Drug	Effect of Interaction
Ergot alkaloids	Increased ergot levels[a]
Fluconazole	Increase saquinavir levels
Food	Fat meal improves bioavailability
Grapefruit juice	Increases saquinavir levels
Ketoconazole	Increase saquinavir levels 3× (advantage)
Lovastatin	Risk of myopathy[a]
Midazolam	Increased midazolam levels[a]
Phenobarbital	Decreased saquinavir levels
Phenytoin	Decreased saquinavir levels
PI and NNRTIs	
Amprenavir	APV levels decrease 32%, SQV decrease 19%—Fortovase 800 mg tid + APV 800 mg tid
Delavirdine	SQV levels increase 5×, DLV no effect—Fortovase 800 mg tid + DLV standard dose
Efavirenz	SQV levels decrease 62%, EFV decrease 12%—combination not recommended
Indinavir	IDV unchanged, SQV increased 4–7×—data inadequate
Lopinavir/ritonavir	LPV levels unchanged, SQV levels increased 3.5×—Fortovase 800 mg bid + LPV/r 400/100 mg bid
Nelfinavir	NFV levels increase 20%, SQV levels increase 3–5×—NFV standard dose, Fortovase 800 mg tid or 1200 mg bid
Nevirapine	SQV levels decreased 25%, NVP no effect—no data
Ritonavir	SQV levels increase 20×—SQV (Invirase or Fortovase) 400 mg bid + RTV 400 bid or SQV (Fortovase) 1600 mg qd + RTV 100 mg qd
Rifabutin	Decreased saquinavir levels by 40%[a]
Rifampin	Decreased saquinavir levels by 80%[a]
Sildenafil	Increased sildenafil levels—do not exceed 25 mg/48 hr
Simvastatin	Risk of myopathy[a]
St. John's wort	Decreased SQV levels[a]
Terfenadine (Seldane)	Increased terfenadine levels with possible ventricular arrhythmias[a]
Triazolam	Increased triazolam levels[a]

Serostim (growth hormone)—drug interactions have not been studied

Sulfonamides

Barbiturates	Increased thiopental levels
Cyclosporine	Decreased cyclosporine levels with sulfamethazine
Digoxin	Decreased digoxin levels with sulfasalazine

Table 40. (continued)

Drug	Effect of Interaction
Food	Decreased absorption
Hypoglycemic, oral	Increased hypoglycemic effect of sulfonylurea
Methotrexate	Increased methotrexate levels
Monoamine oxidase inhibitors	Increased phenelzine levels with sulfisoxazole
Phenytoin	Increased phenytoin levels except with sulfisoxazole
Warfarin (coumadin)	Increased hypoprothrombinemia

Tetracycline

Drug	Effect of Interaction
Alcohol	Decreased doxycycline levels in alcoholics
Antacids	Decreased tetracycline levels with antacids containing Ca^{++}, Al^{++}, Mg^{++}, and $NaHCO_3$
Antidepressants, tricyclic	Localized hemosiderosis with amitriptyline and minocycline
Anti-diarrhea agents	Agents containing kaolin and pectin or bismuth subsalicylate, decreased tetracycline levels
Barbiturates	Decreased doxycycline levels[a]
Bismuth subsalicylate (Pepto-Bismol)	Decreased tetracycline levels[a]
Carbamazepine (Tegretol)	Decreased doxycycline levels[a]
Contraceptives, oral	Decreased contraceptive effect (? significance)
Digoxin	Increased digoxin levels (10% of population)
Food (dairy products)	Decreased absorption except with doxycycline
Iron, oral	Decreased tetracycline levels and decreased iron effect; give 3 hr before
Laxatives	Agents containing Mg^{++} decrease tetracycline levels
Lithium	Possible increased lithium toxicity (single case)
Methotrexate	Increased methotrexate levels
Methoxyflurane anesthesia (Penthrane)	Possibly lethal nephrotoxicity[a]
Milk	Decreased absorption of tetracycline[a] Does *not* apply to doxycycline or minocycline
Molindone	Decreased tetracycline levels
Phenformin	Decreased doxycycline levels[a]
Phenytoin	Decreased doxycycline levels
Rifampin and rifabutin	Possible decreased doxycycline levels
Theophylline	Increased theophylline levels
Warfarin (Coumadin)	Increased hypoprothrombinemia
Zinc	Decreased tetracycline levels[a]

Trimethoprim

Drug	Effect of Interaction
Amantadine	Increased levels of both drugs
Azathioprine	Leukopenia
Cyclosporine	Increased nephrotoxicity[a]

Table 40. (continued)

Drug	Effect of Interaction
Dapsone	Increased levels of both drugs; increased methemoglobinemia
Digoxin	Possible increased digitalis levels
Phenytoin	Increased phenytoin levels
Rifampin	Decreased trimethoprim levels
Thiazide diuretics	Possible increased hyponatremia with concomitant use of amiloride with thiazide diuretics
Trimethoprim-sulfamethoxazole	
Amantadine	Amantadine toxicity with delirium
Ganciclovir	Increased neutropenia
Mercaptopurine	Decreased mercaptopurine levels[a]
Methotrexate	Megaloblastic anemia[a]
Phenytoin	Increased phenytoin levels[a]
Procainamide	Increased procainamide levels
Warfarin (coumadin)	Increased hypoprothrombinemia
Trimetrexate	
Acetaminophen	Increased trimetrexate levels
AZT	Increased bone marrow suppression
Cimetidine	Increased trimetrexate levels
Erythromycin	Increased trimetrexate levels
Fluconazole	Increased trimetrexate levels
Ketoconazole	Increased trimetrexate levels
Rifampin, rifabutin	Decreased trimetrexate levels
Vancomycin	
Aminoglycosides	Increased nephrotoxicity and possible increased ototoxicity[a]
Amphotericin B	Increased nephrotoxicity
Cisplatin	Increased nephrotoxicity
Digoxin	Decreased digoxin levels

Adapted from Drug Information for the Health Care Professional. USP DI 21st edition. Micromedex, Englewood CA 2001, p 1–3451.
[a] Concurrent use should be avoided if possible.

Table 41. Financial Assistance Programs

Drug	Program	Contact
Abacavir (Ziagen)	Patient assistance	800-722-9294
Acyclovir (Zovirax)	Patient assistance[a]	800-722-9294
Albendazole	Microsporidosis—available from GlaxoSmithKline	888-825-5249
Amprenavir (Agenerase)	Patient assistance	800-722-9294
Atovaquone (Mepron)	Patient assistance[a]	800-722-9294
Azithromycin (Zithromax)	Patient assistance[a]	800-646-4455
AZT (Retrovir)	Patient assistance[a]	800-722-9294
Cidofovir (Vistide)	Patient assistance[a]	800-445-3235
Ciprofloxacin (Cipro)	Patient assistance[a]	800-998-9180
Clarithromycin (Biaxin)	Patient assistance[a]	800-688-9118
Clindamycin	Patient assistance[a]	800-242-7014
Clotrimazole	Patient assistance[a]	800-998-9180
Daunorubicin	Patient assistance[a]	800-226-2056
D4T (stavudine, Zerit)	Patient assistance[a]	800-272-4878
ddl (Videx) (didanosine)	Patient assistance[a]	800-272-4878
ddC (Hivid) (Zalcitabine)	Patient assistance[a]	800-282-7780
Efavirenz (Sustiva)	Patient assistance	
EPO (Procrit)	Patient assistance[a]	800-553-3851
Fluconazole (Diflucan)	Patient assistance[a]	800-646-4455
Foscarnet (Foscavir)	Patient assistance[a]	800-488-3247
Ganciclovir (IV and oral)	Patient assistance[a]	800-282-7780
G-CSF (Neupogen)	Patient assistance[a]	
GM-CSF (Leukine)	Patient assistance[a]	800-321-4669
Indinavir	Patient assistance[a]	800-850-3430
Interferon		
Roferon	Patient assistance[a]	800-443-6676
Intron	Product information and Patient assistance[a]	800-521-7157
Itraconazole (Sporonox)	Patient assistance[a]	800-652-6227
Ketoconazole (Nizoral)	Patient assistance[a]	800-652-6227
Lamivudine (3TC)	Patient assistance[a]	800-722-9294
Lopinavir	Patient assistance[a]	800-659-9050
Megestrol (Megace)	Patient assistance[a]	800-272-4878
Nevirapine	Patient assistance[a]	800-274-8651
Nystatin	Patient assistance[a]	800-272-4878
Oxandrolone (Oxandrin)	Patient assistance[a]	800-741-2698
Pyrimethamine	Patient assistance[a]	800-722-9294

Table 41. (continued)

Drug	Program	Contact
Rifabutin	Patient assistance[a]	800-242-7014
Ritonavir (Norvir)	Patient assistance[a]	800-659-9050
Saquinavir (Invirase, Fortovase)	Patient assistance[a]	800-282-7780
Serostim (growth hormone)	Patient assistance and annual $36,000 cap	888-628-6673
Streptomycin	Free supply (Pfi)	800-254-4445
Thalidomide	Availability from STEPS (Celgene)	888-423-5436
Trimetrexate	Patient assistance[a]	800-321-4669
Zidovudine (AZT, Retrovir)	Patient assistance[a]	800-722-9294

[a] Usual requirements are lack of prescription drug insurance (including state plans and Ryan White funds) usually accompanied with income/asset criteria.

10—Major Complications of HIV Infection

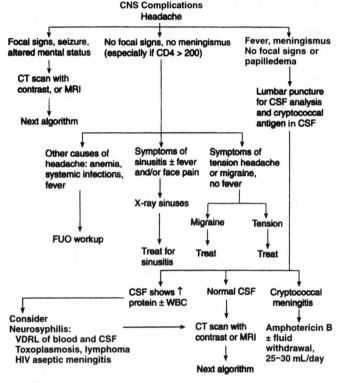

Figure 3. Headache. CT, computed tomography; MRI, magnetic resonance imaging; CSF, cerebrospinal fluid; FUO, fever of unknown origin; WBC, white blood cell count; VDRL, venereal disease research laboratory.

Table 42. Central Nervous System Infection: Differential Diagnosis

Agent	Course	Frequency Setting	Typical Findings	Diagnosis
Toxoplasmosis	Acute	Common: 3–10% of all AIDS patients; 20–35% of AIDS patients with CD4 <100 plus positive serology without prophylaxis	*Mental status*—reduced; *temp*: fever; *scan*: ring-enhanced lesions with mass effect and usually multiple lesions widely distributed; *CSF*: increased protein and 0–40 monos: nl 25%	Typical clinical and scan findings: Response to empiric treatment with clinical improvement in ≤1 wk or scan improvement in 2 wk; IgG serology positive in 85–95%
Lymphoma	Typically subacute	3% of all AIDS patients CD4 <100	*Mental status*—variable; *temp*: afebrile; *scan*: solid-enhanced lesions with mass effect; *location*: periventricular, multiple in 60%; *CSF*: increased protein and 0–100 monos: nl 40%	Typical clinical and scan findings ± failure to respond to empiric treatment of toxoplasmosis; PCR for Epstein-Barr virus in CSF
PML	Subacute	1–3% of all AIDS patients, CD4 <200	*Mental status*—alert; *temp*: afebrile; *scan*: punctate, nonenhanced discrete multifocal lesions without mass effect; *location*: subcortical white matter; *CSF*: normal	Typical clinical and scan findings; stereotactic biopsy-antibody to SV40; characteristic inclusions in oligodendrocytes; PCR for JC virus (40–50% false negative)
Cryptococcal	Acute, subacute, or chronic	Common: 8–12% of all AIDS patients; CD4 <100 median—20	*Mental status*—alert; *temp*: fever; *scan*: no focal lesions; *location*: basal ganglia; *CSF*: increase protein, 0–100 monos, decreased glucose, nl in 20%	CSF: cryptococcal antigen and positive culture: blood: cryptococcal antigen positive in >90% with meningitis

Table 42. (continued)

Agent	Course	Frequency Setting	Typical Findings	Diagnosis
AIDS dementia complex (ADC)	Subacute or chronic	20–30% of all AIDS patients; CD4 <100	*Mental status*—alert; *temp:* afebrile; *scan:* atrophy and ill-defined changes of deep white matter; *location:* deep white matter; CSF: increased protein and 5–10 monos. Beta-2 microglobulin >3 mg/L; nl 40%	Neuropsychiatric tests show subcortical dementia combined with typical scan; mini-mental is insensitive
CMV encephalitis	Acute	1–2% of all AIDS patients; CD4 <50	*Mental status*—delirious; *temp:* afebrile; hyponatremia caused by CMV adrenalitis; *scan:* periventricular infection; CSF: increased protein, decreased glucose, 10–1000 monos	CSF: Cultures negative, PCR usually positive; typical clinic setting and scan: empiric anti-CMV therapy
Neurosyphilis	Asymptomatic Meningeal Tabes dorsalis General paresis Meningovascular Ocular	0.5%; any stage	Variable with stage CSF: increased protein, 5–100 monos ± VDRL	Blood VDRL and FTA-ABS positive + typical CSF changes; CSF VDRL + in 65%; specificity—100%
Tuberculosis	Chronic	0.5–1%	*Mental status*—reduced; *temp:* fever; *scan:* intracerebral enhancing lesions in 50–70%; CSF: increased protein, 5–2000 monos; decreased glucose, nl 5–10%	Chest x-ray; culture positive from any site; CSF culture positive in 20%; PPD variable

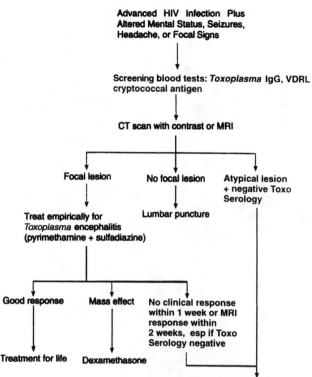

Figure 4. CNS evaluation. CT, computed tomography; MRI, magnetic resonance imaging; FA, fluorescent antibody; PML, polymorphonuclear leukocyte.

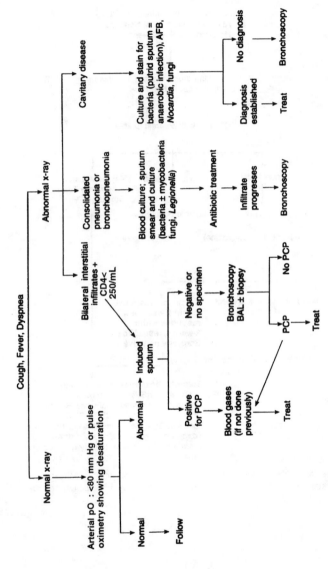

Figure 5. Pulmonary complications.

Table 43. Pulmonary Infection: Differential Diagnosis

Agent	Course[a]	Frequency Setting	Typical Findings	Diagnosis[b]
Bacteria				
S. pneumoniae	Acute	Common, all stages HIV infection	Lobar or bronchopneumonia ± pleural effusion	Sputum GS, quellung, culture, blood culture
H. influenzae	Acute	Moderately common; all stages HIV infection	Bronchopneumonia	Sputum GS and culture
Gram-negative bacilli	Acute	Uncommon, except with nosocomial infection, neutropenia, chronic antibiotic exposure, or late stage disease (especially P. aeruginosa)	Lobar or bronchopneumonia, cavity	Sputum GS and culture
Legionella[c]	Acute	Unusual except in epidemic and endemic areas	Bronchopneumonia multiple noncontiguous segments	Culture on selective media and urinary antigen (L. pneumophila, type 1)
S. aureus	Acute	Uncommon except with influenza or tricuspid valve endocarditis with septic emboli in drug abusers	Bronchopneumonia or multiple nodules ± cavitation	Blood cultures (endocarditis), sputum, GS, and culture
Nocardia[c]	Chronic or asymptomatic	Uncommon: late stage HIV	Nodule or cavity	Sputum or FOB; GS, modified AFB stain and culture
Mycobacteria tuberculosis (MTB)[c]	Chronic, subacute, or asymptomatic	Risk with HIV is ↑ 100-fold; all stages—mean CD4 is 200–300/mm³; extrapulmonary TB common	Variable: Focal infiltrates, reticular, cavity disease, hilar adenopathy, lower and middle lobe involvement common, pleural effusion	Sputum AFB stain and culture; induced sputum or bronchoscopy

Table 43. (continued)

Agent	Course[a]	Frequency Setting	Typical Findings	Diagnosis[b]
M. avium complex (MAC)	Chronic	Infrequent CDR <50; disseminated MAC with bacteremia and no pulmonary involvement is more common	Variable	Recovery in sputum or FOB: Must distinguish from MTB (DNA or radiometric culture technique); MA may colonize airways without causing pulmonary disease
M. kansasii	Chronic or asymptomatic	Uncommon: Late-stage HIV, CD4 <50	Cavity disease, nodule, cyst, infiltrate	Recovery in sputum or FOB
Fungi				
Pneumocystis[c]	Subacute or chronic	Very common in late stages of HIV infection (CD4 <200; median CD4 130 without prophylaxis, 30 with prophylaxis)	Interstitial infiltrates; negative x-ray in 10–30%; also has ↑LDH (90%), ↓pO2 (95%), ↓ pulse oximetry, ↓ diffusing capacity	Cytopath of induced sputum or FOB, yield with induced sputum 40–80% (average 60%) and depends on quality assurance, yield with FOB BAL: >95%
Cryptococcus	Chronic, subacute, or asymptomatic	Moderately common: Advanced HIV infection; median CD4 is 50; 80% have cryptococcal meningitis	Nodule, cavity, diffuse, or nodular infiltrates	Sputum or FOB stain and culture, serum usually shows cryptococcal antigen, LP indicated
Histoplasma capsulatum[c]	Chronic or subacute	Uncommon outside endemic area, usually advanced HIV infection with disseminated histoplasmosis—median CD4 is 50	Diffuse or nodular infiltrates, nodule, focal infiltrate, cavity, hilar adenopathy	Sputum or FOB stain and culture; serum and/or urine antigen assay positive in 80–90%; highest yield with culture: Marrow

Organism	Onset	Epidemiology	Radiographic findings	Diagnosis
Coccidioides immitis[c]	Chronic or subacute	Uncommon outside endemic area, median CD4 is 50	Diffuse or nodular infiltrates, focal infiltrate, cavity, hilar adenopathy	Sputum or FOB stain and culture, serology
Candida	Chronic or subacute	Common isolate, rare cause of pulmonary disease, median CD4 is 50	Bronchitis, rare cause of pulmonary infiltrate	Recovery in sputum or analysis of respiratory specimens is meaningless, should have histological evidence of invasion on biopsy
Aspergillus	Acute or subacute	Up to 4% of patients with advanced HIV infection, corticosteroids and neutropenia (ANC <500/mm^3)	Focal infiltrate, cavity often pleural-based; changes on CT scan or x-ray are often typical	Sputum stain and culture: False-positive and false-negative cultures common; most reliable are positive stain in typical setting with characteristic scan or x-ray or biopsy evidence of tissue invasion
Virus CMV	Subacute or chronic	Common isolate, rare cause of pulmonary disease; advanced HIV infection with median CD4 <20	Interstitial infiltrates	Yield of CMV by cytopath or culture with FOB is 20–50%; diagnosis of CMV pneumonitis requires CMV by biopsy or CMV plus progressive disease *and no alternative pathogen*
Influenza[c]	Acute	Influenza is common; influenza pneumonia is rare; any stage of HIV infection frequency and course similar to that seen with patients without HIV infection	URI, pharyngitis, bronchitis—most common. Bronchopneumonia or interstitial infiltrates are rare except with bacterial superinfection	Culture or rapid stain for influenza virus with respiratory secretions; physician diagnosis based on clinical symptoms in a flu epidemic has a sensitivity of 85%

Table 43. (continued)

Agent	Course[a]	Frequency Setting	Typical Findings	Diagnosis[b]
Miscellaneous Kaposi's sarcoma	Chronic or asymptomatic	Moderately common in patients with cutaneous KS	Interstitial, alveolar, or nodular infiltrates; hilar adenopathy pleural effusions; gallium scan usually negative	FOB: Endobronchial lesion often seen; yield with FOB biopsy of parenchymal lesion is only 10–30%
Lymphoma	Chronic or asymptomatic	Uncommon but may be presenting site	Interstitial, alveolar, or nodular infiltrates; cavity, hilar adenopathy, pleural effusions	FOB: Yield with transbronchial or lymph node biopsy is variable; may need transmediastinal or open lung biopsy or alternative site usually required
Lymphocytic interstitial pneumonia (LIP)	Chronic or subacute	Uncommon in adults CD4 often >200	Diffuse reticular infiltrates, focal infiltrate	FOB: Yield with biopsy is 30–50%; open lung biopsy often required

[a] Course: Acute—symptoms evolve over days; subacute—symptoms evolve over 2–6 wk; chronic—symptoms evolve over >4 wk.
[b] Diagnosis: Expectorated sputum for bacterial culture should have cytological screening to show predominance of PMN; Gram stain (GS) and quellung (if Gram stain suggest S. pneumoniae). Induced sputum is usually reserved for patients with nonproductive cough and suspected PCP or M. tuberculosis. Fiberoptic bronchoscopy (FOB) assumes bronchoalveolar lavage specimen (BAL) ± touch preps, bronchial washings, bronchial brush, or transbronchial biopsy. Detection of fungi includes stains (KOH and/or Gomori's methenamine-silver stain) and culture (Sabouraud's agar); Candida spp. grow on conventional bacteria media. Detection of viruses includes cytopathology for inclusions (herpes viruses—CMV, HSV, VZV); FA for HSV and rapid tests for influenza (see Med Lett 1999;41:121).
[c] Detection of these organisms in respiratory secretions is essentially diagnostic of disease. Other organisms may be contaminants, colonizing mucosal surfaces or commensals.

Table 44. Oral Lesions: Differential Diagnosis

Condition	Clinical Features	Diagnosis
Candidiasis (thrush)	White plaques on inflamed base; CD4 count <300 ± antibiotics	Usually a clinical diagnosis; KOH or Gram stain shows yeast and pseudomycelia
Oral hairy leukoplakia	White hairlike projections usually on lateral surface of tongue; CD4 count <300	Usually a clinical diagnosis and often mistaken for thrush. Biopsy shows hairlike projections with EBV by FA stain
Herpes simplex	Small painful vesicles on inflamed base, especially palate or gingiva; any CD4 count but chronic and severe with <100	Usually a clinical diagnosis in patient with history of "cold sores." Smear will show multinucleate giant cells with HSV by FA stain and culture
Aphthous ulcers	Crops of painful ulcers on mucosal surface; any CD4 count	Negative evaluation for HSV, CMV, VZV
Kaposi's sarcoma	Purple or black nodules usually on palate or gingiva; CD4 count <300	Clinical appearance. Biopsy may confirm diagnosis

Table 45. Dysphagia/Odynophagia: Differential Diagnosis

Condition	Clinical Features	Diagnosis
Candida esophagitis	Accounts for 50–70%. Usually has thrush, diffuse esophageal pain, afebrile, CD4 count <100	Usually a presumed diagnosis with odynophagia and thrush Endoscopy—white plaques, brushing or histology shows yeast; culture should not be done except to test for Candida azole resistance
CMV	Accounts for 10–20%. Pain is focal and severe, fever is common. CD4 count <100	Biopsy required for treatment Endoscopy shows one or multiple ulcers; biopsy shows CMV inclusions; culture not recommended
Herpes simplex	Accounts for 2–5%. Usually has oral ulcers, focal pain, fever uncommon, CD4 count <100	Endoscopy shows small confluent ulcers; biopsy shows HSV inclusions, positive FA stain, and culture
Idiopathic (aphthous ulcers)	Accounts for 10–20%. Focal pain, afebrile, CD4 count variable	Negative evaluation for pathogens Endoscopy—appears like CMV

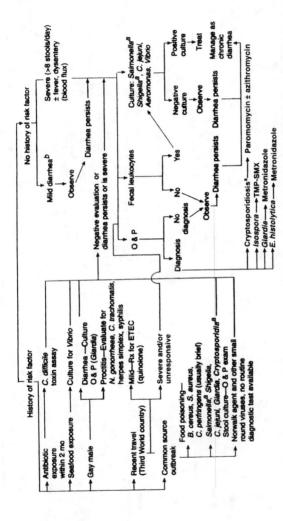

Figure 6. Acute diarrhea with or without fever. [a] Pathogens considered more frequent and/or severe in patients with advanced HIV infection. [b] Most diarrhea is due to medications, anxiety, irritable bowel syndrome, or untreatable viral agents (Norwalk agent, other small round viruses, etc); factors that increase the likelihood of a treatable pathogen are severity of diarrhea, presence of fever, and fecal leukocytes and/or blood.

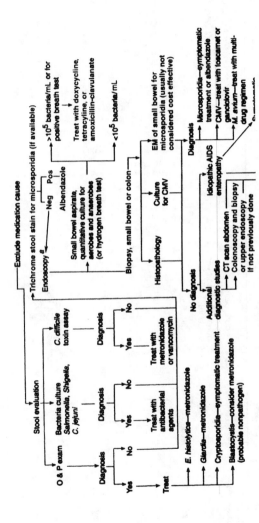

Figure 7. Chronic diarrhea with or without wasting with advanced HIV infection. [a] Lower endoscopy is appropriate as initial endoscopy procedure if there is evidence of colonic disease by symptoms (cramps, dysentery, tenesmus), fecal white blood cells, fecal blood, or CT scan. Upper endoscopy is preferred if there is large volume of diarrhea without fever or cramps and negative fecal WBC exam.

Table 46. Diarrhea: Differential Diagnosis

Agent	Course[a]	Frequency/Setting	Typical Findings	Diagnosis[b]
Bacteria				
Salmonella	Acute or subacute	5–15% of acute diarrheas; any stage of HIV	Enteric fever or gastroenteritis	Blood and stool culture; fecal WBC variable
Shigella	Acute	1–3% of acute diarrheas; any CD4 count	Dysentery (blood and mucus); fever common; colitis	Stool culture; fecal WBC usually present
C. jejuni	Acute	4–8% of acute diarrheas; any CD4 cell count	Stools watery or dysenteric; fever variable; colitis	Stool culture; fecal WBC often present
C. difficile	Acute or chronic	10–15% of acute diarrheas; virtually always with antibiotic exposure, especially clindamycin, ampicillin, or cephalosporins	Stools watery; fever and leukocytosis common; colitis; serum albumin usually low	C. difficile toxin assay; fecal WBC variable
Small bowel overgrowth	Chronic	Frequency unknown	Stools watery; no fever malabsorption	Small bowel aspirate for quantitative culture and/or hydrogen breath test; fecal WBC negative
Mycobacteria M. avium	Chronic	10–20% of chronic diarrheas; CD4 <50	Watery diarrhea; enteritis	Most patients have MAC bacteremia with fever Small bowel biopsy with AFB stain ± culture; fever, abdominal pain

	Acute or Chronic	Epidemiology/CD4	Clinical Features	Diagnosis
Parasites				
Cryptosporidium	Acute or chronic	20-30% of chronic diarrheas CD4 <200	Stools watery, up to 20 L/d usually afebrile, enteritis	Stool AFB or DFA stain: shows typical oocytes; fecal WBC negative
Isospora	Chronic	1-2% of chronic diarrheas: CD4 <100	Stools watery, fever uncommon, enteritis	Stool AFB smear, fecal WBC negative
Microsporidia	Chronic	15-20% of chronic diarrheas; CD4 <50	Stools watery, fever uncommon, enteritis	Trichrome stain of stool to detect microsporidia "gold standard" is EM of small bowel biopsy (or Giemsa stain)
Giardia	Chronic	1-2% of chronic diarrheas; more common in gay men and travelers; any CD4 count	Watery diarrhea ± malabsorption; no fever; symptoms include bloating, flatulence; enteritis	Stool O & P exam: *Giardia* antigen assay
E. histolytica	Chronic or subacute	1-2% of chronic diarrheas more common in gay men and travelers; any CD4 count	Asymptomatic carriage common, especially in gay men; symptoms include bloody stools and fever; colitis	Stool O & P exam: stool shows RBCs; ability of techs to find trophs highly variable—suggest three stool specimens. endoscopy with scraping or biopsy; serology—IFA titer ↑ AFB on stool shows circular organisms larger than *Cryptosporidium*
Cyclospora cayetanensis	Chronic	<1 of chronic diarrheas	Watery diarrhea	
Viruses				
CMV	Chronic or subacute	10-40% of chronic diarrheas; CD4 count <50	Enteritis or colitis; represents disseminated CMV; fever, pain; may cause colonic perforation, acute bleed	Intestinal biopsy to show CMV inclusions ± culture; CMV sometimes seen in absence of inflammation or symptoms

Table 46. (continued)

Agent	Course[a]	Frequency/Setting	Typical Findings	Diagnosis[b]
Enteric viruses	Acute or chronic	15–30% of acute diarrheas; any CD4 count	Enteritis; watery diarrhea	Major agents cannot be detected by clinical labs—astrovirus, adenoviruses, caliciviruses, picobirnavirus
Idiopathic	Chronic	20–30% of chronic diarrheas	Watery diarrhea, small intestinal biopsy shows ↓villus; crypt ratio without ↑intraepithelial lymphocytes	Diagnosis based on typical histological changes and negative studies for microbial cause

[a] Course: Chronic indicates diarrhea for most days during ≥1 mo.

[b] Diagnosis: 1) Stool culture in most labs includes selective media for *Shigella, Salmonella,* and *C. jejuni ± E. coli* 0157. *Aeromonas, Plesiomonas, Yersina,* and *Vibrios.* 2) Preferred test for *C. difficile* is the EIA or tissue culture assay. 3) O & P exam should be done in fresh stool or stool fixed with polyvinyl alcohol. 4) Modified AFB stain detects *Cryptosporidia, Isospora, Cyclospora,* and *M. avium.* 5) Fecal WBC exam distinguishes "inflammatory" and "secretory" diarrheas: A positive result specifically suggests CMV *Salmonella, Shigella, C. jejuni, C. difficile, Yersina, Aeromonas,* or *Vibrio parahemolyticus.* 6) Serology is useful primarily for *E. histolytica* using IFA, which is increased in 85% with amebic colitis. Endoscopy includes proctoscopy, sigmoidoscopy, colonoscopy, and small bowel endoscopy; these are in ascending order of cost and diagnostic utility for unselected AIDS patients and diarrhea. Proctoscopy is preferred for patients with proctitis (usually caused by STDs, including *N. gonorrheae, Chlamydia trachomatis,* herpes simplex, and syphilis); small bowel endoscopy with duodenal biopsy has highest yield in patients with "noninflammatory" chronic diarrhea in late stages of HIV infections; colonoscopy or sigmoidoscopy is preferred in patients with evidence of colitis (i.e., pain, fever, tenesmus, bloody stools, and/or fecal leukocytes).

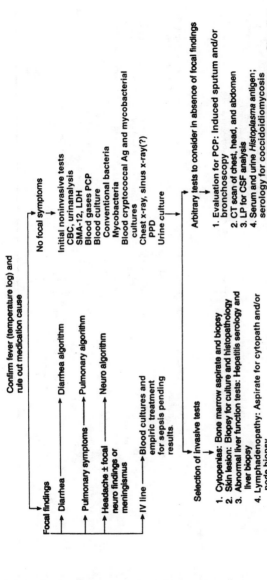

Figure 8. Fever of unknown origin. Most common causes are TB, PCP, disseminated MAC, lymphoma, and/or drug fever.

Table 47. Dermatologic Complications: Differential Diagnosis

Condition	Presentation	Diagnosis
Adverse drug reaction	Red, papular, pruritic rash most common. Less common: Urticaria, erythema multiforme, photosensitivity. Any CD4 count	Response to drug holiday usually adequate unless severe or unresponsive. Association with drugs, especially TMP-SMX, dapsone, nevirapine, delavirdine, or efavirenz
Bacillary angiomatosis	Papules or nodules. Resembles Kaposi's sarcoma. CD4 variable, usually <200	Biopsy: Warthin—starry stain shows B. henselae. Responds to erythromycin
Cryptococcosis	Nodular, ulcerative, or vesicular lesions may resemble HSV, VZV, or molluscum. CD4 <100	Biopsy: Methenamine stain shows yeast
Eosinophilic folliculitis	Pruritic papules and pustules; CD4 <250	Biopsy: Eosinophilic infiltrate in follicular epithelium
Herpes simplex	Vesicles with erythematous base—oral, genital, perirectal, or general cutaneous. Chronicity and severity inversely related to CD4 count	Tzanck prep showing multinucleate giant cells; FA stain and/or culture for HSV ± sensitivity tests in refractory cases
Herpes zoster	Vesicles on erythematous base in dermatomal distribution. Complications are pain, including postherpetic neuralgia, disseminated disease, blindness; any CD4 count	Biopsy. Tzank prep shows multinucleate giant cells. Distinguish from HSV by culture or FA stain
Kaposi's sarcoma	Firm subcutaneous brown-black or purple nodules, any cutaneous site especially face, chest, genitals, extremities	Must distinguish from bacillary angiomatosis. Biopsy
Molluscum contagiosum	Pearly white or flesh colored papules with central umbilication; most common on face and genitals	Usually clinical appearance. EM of scraping of vesicle fluid
Psoriasis	Plaques that are sharply demarcated, especially knees, elbows, scalp, lumbosacral area	Biopsy with histopath may resemble seborrhea or drug eruption
Seborrhea	Erythematous, scaling plaques with indistinct margins, especially scalp, butterfly region of face, ears, hairline, chest, upper back, axilla, groin	Clinical features
S. aureus	Folliculitis ± pruritis, especially trunk, groin, face	Exudate should show typical GPC and grow S. aureus

INDEX

Note: Page numbers in *italics* indicate material presented in figures. Page numbers followed by letter *t* indicate tables.

235